Glimpse of the Afterlife

Near Dear Experiences

Lekatt

Cover Art by Maggie K. S.

Glimpse of the Afterlife

Copyright © 2021 by Leroy Kattein

All rights reserved. No part of this book may be reproduced or transmitted in any form or by any means without written permission of the author.

ISBN

Dedication

This book is dedicated to those
who struggle with life.
May it ease their journey.

Acknowledgment

It took great courage for them to write and post their
experiences. I acknowledge their willingness
to help others by sharing them.

Foreword

This book is a collection of Near Death Experiences. The NDE happens when a trauma stops the heart and causes clinical death. This clinical death can last for only a few minutes, an hour, or more. When the person is revived or returns to life they tell of experiencing a short glimpse of the afterlife. These writings are what they saw and felt in their own words. They were posted anonymously with only first name or initials to my website and blog.

It takes a lot of courage to go public with a near death experience. Some believe they are only dreams or hallucinations. That has been proven wrong with evidence collected by researchers. The near death experience is a real glimpse of a spiritual existence awaiting us all.

Table of Contents

Table of Contents

Notes

Diving into the Shallow End of the Ocean

I'm 44 and last year I broke my neck while diving into the shallow end of the ocean.

Not a recommended recreation. Everything went white and although I realized I had just "bought the farm," the white place seemed very familiar and comfortable.

Below me was my body floating face down in the surf. The irony here is that my business name is Tsunami, which means "great wave." Not being at all concerned with this situation, I had but one regret -- that I didn't get the chance to say goodbye to my children. With that thought I re-entered my body through the back/top of my head, the same place from where I left only moments before.

Now I was aware that I was paralysed and couldn't get out of the water, much less sit up and breath, so I tried to leave my body again from the back of my head. Only now I was stuck inside my body, with the sound of the sand underwater and the realization that the air in my lungs was being used up, I was not at all pleased to find myself in this predicament. I said a quick prayer to Creator to help me out (of my body) but before I knew it, a wave had sat me up on the very sandbar I had just smashed into with my head. I could taste blood. My head felt like a white hot nail had just been hammered into it. I tried to wipe off my mouth and face, but my hand was nowhere near where my brain was trying to convince me it was. The other hand was nowhere in sight either.

This was getting worse by the second and I was beginning to panic (in my head). Then a voice (from who knows where) said, "It's time to use other parts of your brain. Just re-lax and try to touch your finger to your nose. Take your time. You have plenty of brain power in reserve but it needs a little review. Just try to *think* your finger to your nose."

So I did. It took perhaps five minutes of practice and I must have looked like a DWI refugee. But I managed to touch my finger to my nose WITH MY EYES CLOSED. Then I felt the electricity return to my feet and I could wiggle my toes.

So I stood up and walked out of the ocean and walked 1 1/2 miles back to the house, although very slowly and holding my head on the whole way. I broke the atlas (the first vetibrae) clean in half and severely dam-aged the ligament inside of that bone. I also fractured the 7th vertibra or the last neck bone. This kind of accident usually results in death (which I KNOW it did) and my doctor is amazed that I'm around to tell the story.

I've had lucid dreams and out of body experiences and have had what I would consider and abduction senario happen since way back in 1964, way before any of this space stuff was in the media. I've also had my mind spontaneously shut off all internal dialogue and had my awareness expand to encompass the entire universe, without prompting and without drugs.

All of these experiences are gifts that have taken me many years to understand. Breaking my neck and being here to tell you about is also a gift... a gift to tell any who wishes to read about it that there is more than just this body and just this life. Your life is an experience. Enjoy and learn. Don't worry. LOVE!!! -- W.D.

Death by Road Accident

Here is my life's most important experience, first the events leading up to it, my parents report of occurrences while I was away, my NDE, and finally how I feel about it.

Scene: 24/02/82, Newcastle Australia, 6;00 pm, Leaving my optical instrument repair firm to go home to Raymond Terrace, Raining after 3 months Dry, I was driving along the Industrial Highway and slowing to stop at lights where exit road from BHP crosses highway, memory ends.

Medical Info: Stewart's spine was broken L4, I suffered Fractures Basal area, Frontal Lobe, Right eye socket, Right Zygote, all depressed, 6 holes in dura, also spokes of steering wheel and indicator entered throat up into roof of mouth, right upper and lower thorax. Miles suffered a small seat belt bruise.

My Mother Reported that: In the afternoon of 25/02/82 they were in the office of Professor *anonymous* (Professor of Neurosurgery) where the prof. was reporting my death and that they should be grateful, as I would have been a vegetable had I survived, during this conversation a young frightened Nurse came rushing into the office, blurting out "She is alive, she sat up and spoke!," the prof. chastised her for interrupting them 3 times before taking her outside and lecturing her about "dead bodies" moving and making noises, the Nurse was emphatic, She sat up and said: "Don't give me any more Drugs!," at this point my mother took the prof. by one elbow, my father by his and marched them down the corridor to see, they found me in a back corridor where I had apparently been placed so the nurse could remove equipment prior to my transfer to the Morgue, I was in deep coma and breathing, I remained in coma for a further 10 days.

My NDE:
I don't know when in the above events my experience took place. I have no memory of the process of dying or leaving my body. I was moving head first through a dark malstorm of what looked like black boiling clouds, feeling that I was being beckoned to the sides which frightened me, ahead was a tiny dot of bright light which steadily grew and brightened as I drew nearer, I became aware that I must be dead and was concerned for Mum & Dad and my Sister, and somewhat upset with myself as I thought "they will soon get over it" like it was in passing just a fleeting thought as I rushed greedily forward towards this light.

I arrived in an explosion of glorious light
into a room with insubstantial walls,
standing before a man about in his 30's
about 6 foot tall, reddish brown shoulder
length hair and an incredibly neat, short
beard & mo., He wore a simple white robe,
light seemed to emanate from Him and I felt
He had great age and wisdom. He
welcomed me with great Love, tranquility,
Peace (indescribable), no words, I felt "I
can sit at your feet forever and be content,"
which struck me as a strange thing to
think/say/feel, I became fascinated by the
fabric of His robe, trying to figure out how
light could be woven!

He stood beside me and directed me to look
to my left, where I was replaying my life's
less complementary moments, I relived
those moments and felt not only what I had
done but also the hurt I had caused, some of
the things I would have never imagined
could have caused pain, I was surprised that
some things I may have worried about, like
shoplifting a chocolate as a child, were not
there whilst casual remarks which caused
hurt unknown to me at the time were
counted, when I became burdened with
guilt I was directed to other events which
gave joy to others, although I felt unworthy
it seemed the balance was in my favor, I
received great Love.

I was led further into the room, which became a hall and there coming towards me was my Grandfather, he looked younger than I remembered and was without his Hare lip or cleft pallet, but undoubtedly my grandfather, we hugged, he spoke to me and welcomed me, I was moved to forgive him for dying when I was 14 and making me break my promise, to become a Doctor and find a cure for his heart condition, until that moment I had not realized I had been angry at him!

Granddad told me that Grandma was coming soon and he was looking forward to her arrival, I inquired why she was coming soon as she had been travelling from her home in Manchester, to NZ, To Miami for continual summer for a number of years! Granddad told me she had Cancer of the Bowel and was coming soon, Granddad seemed to have no grasp of time when I pressed for how soon. (Grandma was diagnosed 3 months later and died in August, I had upset my mother by telling her about it when I regained consciousness.), after Granddad and I had talked a while he took me further into the room which became a hall again, we approached a group of people whom I started to recognize.

The Person who first welcomed me came
and placed his hand on my shoulder and
turned me towards Him, He said "You must
return, you have a task to perform.," I
wanted to argue, I wanted to stay, I glanced
back at Granddad and was propelled
quickly towards the entrance, at the
threshold all became blackness, nothing, no
awareness.

After: I awoke from my coma slowly, over
several days, half dreamed memories of
familiar voices and glimpses of faces. The
clearest moments were several occasions
where I would awake from deep sleep to
find a nurse with a syringe and I refused
any Drugs, I have no idea why!

I had three lots of surgery to repair my face,
skull, eye socket. Left hospital with Pain,
double vision, anosmia, and damage to 8th
cranial nerve left me with nausea and
disturbed balance. I was for two years angry
at G-d, for sending me back in such
torment, with a task to do with no clues or
instructions, only one thing a clear message
I have no idea how to pass on, which is "It
is time to live according to your Beliefs,
whatever they may be, to put your House in
order, For the End Times are upon us!" This
can't be my task, there was no booming
voice, or any way I know the message got

there. I am also unsure of the identity of the
gatekeeper, no name tag, no introduction!

It took me 5 years as a zombie, before I was
able to rehabilitate myself, I have gainful
employment, formed the Head Injury
Society NZ. in 1987, and am paraded as the
example of how well it is possible to
recover from Acquired Brain Damage.

I still don't know my task, still have pain,
anosmia, diplopia, etc.

That's about it except to say that the
memory of the NDE is more real than what
I did yesterday.

Shalom....Peace & Love

Before Birth Experience

All the near death experiences that I have read involve people passing from the physical to the spiritual. My experience is unique in that I can remember before I was born, coming from the spiritual to the physical. My experience is as follows:

I can remember standing in a dark space, but unlike being in a darkened room, I could see everything around me and the blackness had dimension.

There was another person standing to my right, and like me, he was waiting to be born into the physical world. There was an older person with us who could possibly be a guide, since he stayed with us until we left and answered my questions.

Behind us was a crowd of people, but they weren't clear to our vision like the two people standing next to me. The best illustration I've ever seen that could give you an idea of what the crowd looked like, is in the final scenes of the movie "Ghost", where Patrick walks away to join the other spirits. In front of us and approximately 30 degrees below us, we could see the Earth with the facial images of two couples.

I spoke to the other person next to me
briefly, but I can't remember what was said.
I can remember talking to the older man.
When we communicated, it wasn't with
spoken word but with a form of telepathy.
We communicated with thought transfer but
we heard the words clearly as if they were
spoken. I asked the older man who the
people were behind us and he replied that
they were waiting to be born but they
weren't ready yet. I asked him what was that
in front of us and he replied that what we
were looking at was Earth. I then asked him
who those people were whose images
appeared on the Earth and he replied that
they were going to be our parents.

I didn't know which parents we were each
going to end up with. The older man
conveyed to us that it was time to go. The
other person standing next to me walked
forward and disappeared from my sight. I
was told that it was my turn and I walked
forward.

Suddenly I found myself lying in a hospital
nursery with other babies around me. I still
had my normal thought processes at this
stage. I noticed three people standing at the
foot of my bed. I immediately recognized
two of them as my parents. They looked
exactly as their image appeared on the
Earth. The other person was my older

brother, but I didn't know this at the time. I remember lying on my back looking around and thinking this must be Earth. I tried to stand up and found I couldn't, since I was now trapped in a baby's body. I can't recall anything before being in the dark space (it's as if I suddenly was).

My father, who knew nothing of my experience, often talked about the first time they came to the hospital to see me. He said I stared so hard at the three of them that he thought my eyes were going to pop out. I was born in 1965 and man wasn't able to view the Earth as I saw it, until they went to the moon. As a child, when I first saw the photos of the Earth taken by the Astronauts from space, it was exactly as I remembered it.

I can also remember, while still in the spiritual, that the physical world seemed as unreal as the spiritual does from the physical perspective.

Your comments on my experience would be welcomed. I only wish I kept a written record of my experience when I was still a child. Up until I was about 13 years old, I could remember everything that was spoken, word for word.

As a child I freely told other children what happened, because I thought it was a purely natural experience for someone to have such an experience. I only learnt of its uniqueness when I could find no one else who had a similar experience and after continually having my experience discounted as imagination by others. Only recently have I come across a couple of NDE examples where people have seen other people being prepared to be born.

I welcome you to put this on your web site if you so desire. I'm now starting to realise that my experience is too unique and precious, not to be shared with others.

Diabetic

Hi. Thank you for this opportunity to talk
about something which has left me quite
disturbed.

I had my NDE just a few nights ago. How
do you convince anyone that this is not "just
a dream"? I KNOW that I went somewhere.
I don't recall a tunnel to get there, I was just
suddenly there -- in a sort of a room. I could
see my deceased grandparents over at the
other side of the room, but they were
talking among themselves as though they
did not think I should be there. There was a
huge book on the ground and when I
opened it there were pictures of many
people who I know have already died. I
accidentally slammed the book shut and
was suddenly terrified that I had ruined
everything by doing this.

When I reopened the book all the people
looked "dead" (pale and still, eyes shut)
which increased my guilt and terror.
Suddenly my grandmother said "Look
again". When I looked back at the book and
started turning the pages all the people had
come back to "life" -- they were moving,
talking and smiling at me.

A woman in the book said "this will change the way you think about life and death". My grandmother said "see, it's not possible for you to ruin anything permanently". I was happy momentarily, but then I heard knocking on a door. The door had a bright light shining behind it and I could see shadows under it as though people were moving around behind it. I knew these people had come for me, but suddenly I remembered my husband, and I desperately wanted to go back to "earth".

I got very upset because I didn't know if I should answer the door and go with the other people, and I didn't know how to get back to my husband. Suddenly I was in a tunnel with a feeling of hurtling very fast like on a roller coaster. All along the way it was as though I was being given all sorts of understanding, wisdom and peace about life and events and other people, but the thoughts were coming so fast that I knew I'd find it hard to grasp them.

It then felt like I "landed" back in my body. My husband was standing next to me asking me what was wrong. I just lay there stunned, totally unable to move or speak and desperately trying (mostly unsuccessfully) to recall the "wisdom" I'd been given. I didn't know whether to laugh or cry and I still don't know whether to classify this journey as good or scary.

It turned out that my blood sugar had dropped to almost zero (I am a diabetic) and it was amazing that I had ever regained consciousness. I'm sure some people will think this was just hallucinations due to abnormal brain chemistry or something or that it was just a dream but I KNOW that it wasn't -- I know it more than I've ever known anything. I've had weird dreams and very low blood sugar many times before and they are NOTHING like this experience. I know that I really went somewhere else.

I still feel shell-shocked by all this. Even though I do feel certain now about life after death and I do feel that something important has happened to me, I'm totally confused about what else I am meant to do or change I wish I could go back "there" and ask a few more questions!! or at least properly remember the wisdom I was given in the tunnel. It was a result of this. hope this feeling of detachment from life on earth will subside.

Thank you very much for the opportunity to share this. S.J.

While Sleeping

Leroy, Hi! I'm finally getting a chance to email you my nde. As I briefly told you in my other email it happened while I was sleeping. I wasn't sick or injured or anything.

I was having a dream that I was supervising my class on the playground. I'm a teacher. But it wasn't our playground and I didn't know the children. It wasn't any playground I had seen before. Very quickly, I left the playground and was on my bed laying down. I remember thinking how did I get here. As I thought that, my feet started to lift up off the bed, then my head and eventually my whole body was floating and rising. I was weirded out at first then liked it and felt really happy and thought it was fun.

As I began to wonder what was going on I realized and said to myself "Hey I'm dying." I answered my own question. I now recall a figure being with me. I remember it being at the right-hand foot of the bed. That memory came recently. As I realized I was dying I went into a dark area which quickly turned into a tunnel. I began to move up it very quickly.

I was moving at a left-hand angle. There were lights spinning around me as I ascended. At the end of the tunnel there was a very bright light. It got bigger as I got closer to it. I felt very happy, very light and had a cool feeling about me. It was like being in cool water. I knew I was a light also. There was some kind of music or sound as I ascended.

About 1/2 way up I stopped. I started to feel like I wasn't ready to go. Strong thoughts of my husband came. I was upset because he didn't know I was going. I didn't like leaving without telling him. As I thought about him I saw him and felt that I couldn't go because he still needed me.

At the same time I thought about how much I liked being there and how nice it would be to stay. I thought of a soulfriend of mine and if I stayed my spirit could visit him or others anytime I wanted to. I felt very safe like I was home. That was me, not my earth self. I didn't want to leave. I felt complete peace and love.

The thoughts of my husband were very strong and were pulling me downwards. Just like that I woke up in my bed. I was crying and very disoriented. Everything felt and seemed foreign to me. My body felt heavy and awkward, but I still had the cool,

light sensation. It took about an hour for
that to go away. I cried for at least an hour.
I was sobbing and had no idea why. I didn't
like the weight of my body or how hard and
odd things seemed. Everything that was
familiar before wasn't.

I had to readjust to being back in my body
and on earth. It took a long time for me to
do that. Everything was different. I felt
different. Slowly my view on life and love
has changed. I feel like I am evolving
everyday.

My beliefs on religion have changed. I now
believe everything is about love. That God
is love. We all are. We are here to learn this
and to help other people to learn this. I
could go on and on. It's hard to put into
words. Words don't describe well enough.
It's all about feelings.

Thanks for giving me and other people the
opportunity to share these very unique
experiences. It has helped me and has
comforted me. All I hope is that I am doing
the same for people in this life.

Have a Glorious day!!!

K. :)

God is Great

I had my "experience" 6 1/2 years ago, four days prior to my 32nd birthday. I was alone at my office on a Saturday, April 3, 1993. I had experienced terrible headaches for about ten days. I was a trial attorney and I had just completed a major trial. I was drafting a brief for another, and preparing for five other trials in the next three months.

Without warning a blood vessel in my brain ruptured and I was flown by helicopter to Wash. D.C. Hosp. Ctr. in very critical condition. I lost conciousness in the helicopter and I was in a coma for five days.

All that I remember was suddenly being "transported" to a very peaceful place; a feeling of calm overcame me. Suddenly, in front of me, were four people who I knew had passed away over the last 14 years. They were all lined up in front of me, as if to welcome me, when a very calming male voice said "Go Back...it's not your time yet."

My next clear memory is almost 7 weeks later, when they took me off my anti-seizure medication. Since that day I have been unable to return to my practice, and many

bad things have happened to me such as
losing my career and my marriage, but all I
have to do is think of that day and what was
said to me by, I believe God, and I am
suddenly calm, and unconcerned because I
know where I am going and I know what's
ahead of me.

What is Death?

I was in my living room looking in the
mirror, my right eye couldn't focus on my
reflection, I kept blinking and blinking
trying to get it to focus. I felt numbing
going through the right side of my face
leading to the top of my head. My breathing
became short, and it was like there was no
oxygen in the air, my chest squeezed tight;
everything went black and I fell.

Two hours later I woke up. I broke the glass
table I landed on with my back. I know God
made sure no pieces went in my back. I
thought I actually slept there all night. I
thought to myself why would I sleep here
on the floor? I then realized I had passed
out. At the time I thought it was a lack of
iron. I did not realize that I had a minor
stroke.

Later, talking to doctors I realize it. When I
was passed out it seemed like seconds, and
then I woke up. I looked at the clock and
noticed that I had been lying on the floor for
two hours. I didn't go to the doctors at first
because I figured I just passed out no big
deal.

The second time this happened I felt it coming because my right eye seen only black. I could hardly run I was so weak. My heart was beating out of my chest, "really hard" and erratic. My breath was short and rapid. I jumped into bed and figured if I was going to pass out let it be in bed this time. I waited to pass out but my heart was beating so hard I thought it was really going to pop out of my chest. I listened to it as it went boom, boom then stopped all together; then it came back and beat really fast and hard then stopped again. This went on for like five minutes, more erratic heart beats till finally my heart stopped.

I didn't feel any pain anymore. No numbness. What was really weird, I didn't breath anymore. I just lay there thinking okay what now? I didn't realize that I was dead. When I landed on the bed, a pillow was halfway across one eye on my face and I tried to push it off because it was bothering me. I lifted my arm and noticed as I attempted to push the pillow off of my head my arm went right through it. I couldn't believe what had happened so I tried again. This time it really scared me. I lifted my head, which I thought, was my physical head up to try and escape dealing with this, and I saw my leg jump "my physical leg" from nerves. I felt the flesh

get cold. Once in a while my whole
physical flesh jerked and jumped.

Then I started to see through the walls. I
could see through the pillow with both eyes
"still thinking physical". I saw this small
black image hovering over the pillow
looking straight into my eyes; it kept
looking in a eager and greedy way and I
could hear what it was thinking. It was
waiting for me to leave my body.

This figure reminded me of a half human
and frog being, it stood like a frog. Its face
was mutilated. Its eyes were so black you
fell into them as you looked into them. I
screamed at it I don't belong to you I belong
to God! I belong to Jesus!! I finally realized
I was dead. I started to cry but I felt no tears
roll down my face. I just kept crying out I
belong to you, God. I belong to you, Jesus!
There was no response. My life passed by
me as I layed there. I thought of all the
times I sinned and all the times I was good
which were very few.

I kept repeating these words: "I don't want
to die". I waited for God to talk to me, but
there was no response. The demon left my
side after I mentioned Jesus' name, but
Jesus did not come to get me. I was alone. I
didn't see any tunnels. I guess because I
refused to accept my death. I stopped saying

I don't want to die and just cried. I cried so
much that I went into a deep depression.
My soul felt heavy on the bed. I knew at
that point, I did not give my life to God
after all. My life was all a lie.

I just thought to myself, I deserve to go to
hell, I was a filthy sinner. I don't deserve to
go to heaven. It came to a point where I just
gave up. I didn't care anymore. I couldn't
cry, because I was cried out, and God and
Jesus had every right to ignore me because
that's what I did to them all of my life. I
knew, not only was, my flesh dead but so
was my soul.

I was in total despair. I kept hearing my
mom's voice say: "you have to really give
your life to God." "You have to really
except Jesus as your Lord and Savior." I
didn't and it was too late. The last words I
said were I deserve this. For, at least, it
seemed like hours I lay there like a zombie.
Then all of a sudden: these words came out
of me. "Father why hast thou forsaken me"?
Now let me make this clear, I never read the
bible and never cared at all about what it
said.

It was repeated one more time and I was
just laying listening to this voice coming
out of my souls mouth. My whole soul felt
peace and love. Inside my physical stomach

I felt a snap way deep down inside. A warm
feeling ran through my body like electricity.
I jumped out of bed and started running all
over the house I knocked things over
running for about 15 minutes. I kept saying
thank you Jesus for having mercy on
meâ€¦â€¦ Finally I stopped running and
thought of what just happened? I knew it
was the mercy of God that I was living
again.

My heart felt brand new, its beat was soft
and smooth. I looked at the clock to see
how long I was dead and I was dead for
about 1 hour. Maybe more. I am perfectly
heathly to this day. I have given my life to
Jesus â€¦. I thank him for the gift of life he
gave me on that day. My advice to you is:
love is the answer. God is love.

I died when I was 21 in 1991 that was the
day I truly gave my life to Jesus. I pray that
this message will reach those who don't
believe that there is a life after death. I pray
that they hear these words not only in the
flesh but in the spirit.

Thank you for your time and May God
Bless you
With Peace and Love in Jesus' name Amen.

Diana

(What a beautiful NDE. No matter what the belief system or doctrine one holds to be true. It still comes out: "Love is the answer. God is Love.)

My Death Experience

My NDE happened Feb. 10, 1997, I was blown up in an explosion, my eardrums were blown out and my arm was missing, my left eye was full of darkness. I remember getting medical attention in the field. Nothing after that

My experience started out with a slide show of various scenes, these flashed along at such a high speed, in a conscience state they would make no sense. In my state, I not only saw the scenes but experienced the complete "feelings and emotions" that EVERYONE felt. Example: I was walking with a group of people looking for food, I felt the hunger and desperation of the whole tribe, I was walking in a hot, dusty place, hanging on to life, driven to find water and food.

Another example was during a trench war, the scenery looked like WWI. I felt the horror, the death of those around me, the fear of everyone and even the enemies horror in what they were doing. Another scene I wore a blue uniform, with white pants and white crossed shirt, I remember feeling if I stopped I would die, the road was full of snow, a long line of soldiers were marching with me. Horses lay frozen on the side of the road with their riders frozen to them. I felt utter defeat, and despair. I saw many of these strange scenes, some I still don't get.

The next stage was the dark shape void; figures that were totally dark flew around me. They adsorbed all light and were pestering me. I could not see any details other than a void. These scared me.

I then found myself in a corridor, or tunnel, the first thing I thought was, wow, this is kinda neat what is this. I remember feeling the fog that was in the corridor, it was a fog I put my hands in and it felt like nothing. I noticed I was floating along. My body was floating at an angle my head was first. The fog was strange it moved in a circular pattern, basically circles, the fog lined this whole corridor. I noticed on the sides flashing lights like I was in the clouds and it was lightning. The electrical discharges were colored. I saw them flashing in the fog; when I traveled along the corridor I saw that the colored flashes came just before a person entered the corridor. I couldn't make out details, they always moved forward faster than me towards the opening, which was a yellowish light like the sun.

I floated along slowly, I would float in the background. At one point I would see other people greeting the other floaters in the corridor, they hugged and held hands and some walked hand in hand towards the light. I did not recognize anyone. I asked a lot of questions, but it was strange, I thought of the question in my mind, but they were answered before I thought of them? I started to panic, I realized this was death, I started to get scared, "what was happening to me," at that moment a boy came through the tunnel fog. He was probably 12, (I have no idea who it was) he smiled and waved to me. All my fear then disappeared.

I floated in this place for I don't know how long. I asked "God" what my purpose in life was and what am I supposed to do. I told the entity, I didn't want to leave, I was scared. I was told my purpose would be revealed to me, so far it has not been revealed. I also was told I would receive some type of gift, or special ability, I do not know what this would be too. This whole episode was full of such clarity and emotion its beyond description.

The next thing I remember, is various hospital staff voices, and someone telling me my brother was here. I was in the critical burn ward, on life support at a

Hospital. I could communicate only by typing Morse Code in my father's hand, (we are both Ham radio hobbyist). I remember thinking I must be in bad shape; they were crying, a priest was there. So they would not cry, I typed in morse code, as a joke, "Does anyone want to order a Pizza," they realized then I was ok.

That was 2 years ago, I will never forget that day. My life has been very hard since that time. My financial status was erased and I spent my first winter, without running water, or heat. Since then I have become bitter with God, I had a life, it's gone now, I lost my career, my home, my savings, everything.

I was very athletic and was a martial arts instructor, and was into body building, I lost a lot. But, I will never forget this experience, I do not know what is in store for me, if God blessed me, or if he is using me to be an example for others to look at, and feel blessed they are not me.

So far I do not feel gifted, or have not felt anything special. For those of you reading this that might think: "this is another religious person shoving a belief down my throat," well, I am not. I am probably more cynical and bitter towards religion now then ever in my life.

However, this experience was something
that I cannot describe fully in words. This
experience I might not ever understand, but
maybe by posting on this board, someone
who went through the same experience
might know others did too. Until then, I feel
utterly hopeless, and wonder every day if it
would have been better to have traveled into
the light, and never have returned back.

SD

I left my Heart in Heaven

I used to believe that death was the end.

I used to believe that life on earth was the
only life we had.

What transpired to me will alter the above
statements and allow for the most
wonderful feelings to never end.

Late Fall 1987, I had been in the hospital
for quite a while because of an illness called
"Guillian Barre Syndrome". I was on life-
support, paralyzed from head to toe, in an
excruciating pain. If that wasn't enough they
were some complications. I will spare you
the details of the agony.

The whole experience began when I started
feeling that death was coming, I can still
smell it! That part, to me, is still very
painful to remember. It was a slow and
painful death. One day or night, I couldn't
make the difference at the end, I felt like my
heart and my lungs were going to explode, I
knew it was only a matter of moments.
After that critical period, the pain suddenly
stopped. I opened my eyes to see if the
doctors were in my room, I found it strange
that the pain would suddenly stop. I opened

my eyes and I saw what seemed to be a priest and few other people. I could only see their shadows but I knew he was a religious man and I thought of the others as members of my family. I immediately assumed that the doctors had called my family and a priest (traditions, you know...) for my final moments. The priest had got my attention for some reasons, perhaps because he was very tall, and very attractive for a priest! There was a light coming from behind them, a very bright light. It was blinding me. I thought it was coming from the nurse station. The priest seemed to look at me as if he was saying "It's all right, you can go". I closed my eyes and I let myself go.

In a matter of seconds, I started viewing periods of my life, everything flashing before me as if it was on a reel of film scrolling upwards, really fast. After the viewing, I felt ready to go. I then felt some kind of pressure coming from inside my body and out through my mouth. I knew that was my last breath. Everything went silent. Few moments after that, I felt I was still around, I opened my eyes again to see what was going on and I saw the priest still standing at the foot of my bed with the others. He started communicating with me without talking. He explained what was happening to me. I understood what he was telling me the second he was thinking it.

My questions were answered as I was thinking them. I don't remember if I have communicated with the other beings, but I know that they were there as some kind of followers, or students. I just couldn't believe that only the body dies, I was still able to think, to look, to feel!! I wanted to know more (I have an adventurous mind). He told me I will know more, and that he had been sent to escort me to the light. I was able to see that light coming from behind them, the same light which I thought was coming from the nurse station. He then told me it was time to go. I guess he felt I was insecure, he took my hand and looked at me with such tenderness (if I would have had my heart still, it would have melted for sure) I will never forget his beautiful and deep eyes. I felt his love and compassion, his confidence and his knowledge all at once. His love was filling me with such warmth! I wasn't worried anymore. I trusted him, I even had the impression that I knew him and he knew me.

I then felt some kind of vibrations, and I felt I was being sucked up in a whirling motion, at an incredible speed, into a large dark tunnel. In a matter of maybe (earth time) a few seconds, I found myself on my back, the palm of my hands up and my feet pointing forward. It seemed to be a symbolic position. I remember looking at myself and realizing that I was no longer attached to my body. In my mind, the memory of my body was still fresh so I had the impression to still be in it even though I wasn't. I guess it would be like looking in a mirror and not seeing your reflection.

As we were going through the tunnel, I heard a beautiful music, very soft singing, or more like humming. I felt elevated by the music. I felt peace and comfort. As we reached the light, the feelings became very intense. It was the most beautiful thing I had ever felt! I thought it was such a cool and fascinating experience. I must have asked what it was that I was feeling so strongly coming from the light, because I remember being told that the light is produced by the love of the Divine Master, the Almighty. His love is so strong that it produces a light powerful enough to go through different realms! No matter where you are in his Kingdom, you always feel his love. I felt embraced by the light, I was making one with it, I felt free, I felt very much alive, I felt complete. The feelings are very difficult to describe with words because they are way, way beyond that.

I wish that moment would have lasted for eternity, but for reasons still unknown to me today, I had to come back. As I was in the comfort of the light, I suddenly felt myself

being sucked down in the same fashion I
had gone up. The motion abruptly stopped,
and my soul slowly reentered my body. I
then felt very cold, very very cold, and I
was feeling aches and pains all over again. I
opened my eyes and my suspicions were
confirmed, I was back in my body, in the
hospital room. I didn't understand why I
was back, I wanted to stay in that beautiful
place, I wanted to learn more about it, I
wanted to explore. I wanted to stay with my
dear angel. I was missing him already. I felt
like part of me was missing. I was thinking
about what had just happened and I felt his
hand gently touching my head. I felt
comforted and secure and fell asleep. From
that moment on, my health quickly
improved. The doctors were amazed at my
recovery.

I have talked to my family about what had
happened to me but no one seemed to really
want to discuss it. It is only years later that I
have learned that in fact, at one time, they
thought I was died but I came back. Well it
isn't just a thought to me, I have died and
came back.

I will always feel blessed by the experience
and I'll forever be grateful for what I have
seen, felt and most importantly learned. I
know I will go back when the time is right.

I have to, like the song "I left my heart in
San Francisco", well I left mine in Heaven!

Line
Toronto
Canada

There was No Time, No Fear

Many years ago, after returning home from school, I felt very tired and decided that I had to go to my room to lie down. While lying there, I felt so exhausted and heavy that it was impossible for me to stay awake.

Just before I went into a full sleep, I "felt" myself removed from my body. The best way I can describe this feeling is to say that I was "vacuumed" out -- it was painless. I instantly became aware that I had floated up to the ceiling and was looking down at my body. There was a feeling of confusion about this. But it did not last long. The awareness of realizing I had total knowledge of all existence and the most sublime love radiating through me directed my thoughts away from the body lying on the bed. That was no longer me...even though I knew it used to be me.

There was no time...there was no fear...

I felt that "others" were communicating with me -- even though I did not see anyone. But eyes were not used there. I did not hear anyone. But ears were not used there. These beings were present through an awareness in my mind. We communicated through our minds. We each knew what the other was thinking and feeling.

They were there to instruct, or guide, me. In the time that would have been a heartbeat, if there were such a thing as time, I saw my whole "previous" life flash in front of me as if a movie. Beside being aware of the happenings going on around me, I was also aware of and personally felt the emotions of those I had previously had contact with in my life. Some of it I was not proud of. But I was forgiven. Grace was a gift.

The thought of my family entered my mind....I felt they would be extremely upset if I were to stay in this beautiful place. They would not understand my joy. Even though it would be the future, in the life we now know, I could see my father grieving my death. I decided that I needed to return.

Before returning to the body that I know, I was taught by the helpers that everything would be ok...I would return. And the next time I died I would stay. This knowledge brought me great joy.

Returning into the body that I had left was not as comfortable as leaving it was. If only I could find the words to describe this return....it was if I was "slammed" back. I gasped for air, and felt imprisoned in the body that was mine. Gradually, I became more comfortable in myself.

I was startled by the reality of what had occured. But at the same time, I felt at peace. I believed that I could not share this experience with anyone because of the awareness that others would not understand.

Immediately after this happened, my life changed. I was at peace. I did, and do not, fear death. In fact, I look forward to it! My relationships with others changed also. I am now a person who is very "aware". I know what others are going to say before they say it. I can feel and relate to their fears and sorrows...along with their joys. By looking directly into someone's eyes I know their soul. I have only shared about these abilities with one other person.

People whom I do not know tend to gravitate to me. Especially children. They will come to me and want to be held by me. When their parents attempt to retrieve them, the child will resist and even cry while reaching for me. There is a feeling of love...of sharing energies...which at times can be exhausting: especially if one is needy and is unable to give in return.

I have mixed feelings about my life as it is
now. First, I long to return "home". Second,
I feel like an outsider -- very different from
others. Even though I feel frustrated at
times, because of most people's ignorance
(which is not their fault -- they know no
better) I function well in this life.

It seems that the more time that passes since
this experience, the less I can relate to the
awareness of life never ending and the
experience of total love. In order to
"remember" I must share with others. I must
give the gift of what is most precious.

S.

She's not Breathing

Had a request tonight to write about near death experiences. For those of you who have not personally had a near death experience, you will think I'm telling a tall tale. For those of you who have had one, you will relate, nod your head and smile.

In 1978, I went in for surgery. It was to take less than an hour with no complications expected. All of the others had been a snap, so why not this one. The last I remember, I was asking the Doctor if he had had to much to drink the night before. He squeezed my hand and said: "Put her out".

Surgery lasted nearly three hours, but I lost all track of time. Time means nothing on the other side or so I have been led to believe. I had plenty of time to watch what they were doing and to look through everything that was in that operating room. The blanket they wrapped me in after surgery, was in a device I associated with being a microwave oven. I stayed in it for a while because it was very comfortable and the way it kept the blanket warm was fascinating. There are so many, many packages, instruments, tubes and sterilizing equipment ... I was having a ball! The

things the two Doctors and the surgical
Nurses talked about were very funny and
not at all what I expected them to discuss
during surgery. One of the Nurses was more
concerned with a problem at home. She
kept thinking if they'd just shut up she could
think. And then, surgery was over.

But then ... the Anesthetist began to get
upset. His heart rate jumped awfully high
and he kept saying "She's not breathing!
Breathe damn you, breathe." I watched over
his shoulder for a while and wondered why
they did not cover my body up. He was
patting my cheeks with force and talking to
me like I couldn't hear him. Some of his
language wasn't on the polite side. With the
first breath I was back in my body telling
him I was cold. Within seconds, they had
the blanket wrapped around me and I was
warm as toast.

The Anesthetist came in later that night as
they always do. When I told him I had tried
to breathe for him the first time he told me
to, he asked what I was talking about. I told
him about how he had slapped my face and
cussed because I wasn't breathing. He said I
was just dreaming. I asked about the one
nurse with the problem. I asked him about
different things I'd gone through in the
operating room. I told him several things he
knew I could not have known.

I was in the hospital for nine days, but he
never came back to see me after that first
night. He did finally admit that it startled
him when I did not breathe. He also assured
me that he would not have let me die. He
said he would have done everything and
breathed for me as long as necessary.

That was the first time...

Judy

Birth NDE

Hi!

I am glad that you courageously took that first step of putting your pages on the web! I have bookmarked your site for myself today. I was feeling a little down and lost today, and reading some of the stuff you have in your site has helped me feel much better.

I had a NDE when I was being born. To accept my story, not only does the listener have to accept the possibility of NDE, one also has to believe that remembering one's birth is possible! I didn't remember it consciously until I was about 5, when I started having recurring dreams about it. They were always identical, very clear and intense.

I would see/feel myself swimming around in lovely warm water when suddenly I knew I had to get to the surface, because I was running out of air. I started to frog kick towards the surface, a vaguely lit surface above me. I kicked hard for a minute or so, and then realized that it wasn't getting any closer. It was like I was tied to the bottom somehow. The surface was maddeningly

close, but I could make no progress towards
it. I relaxed then, realizing that I was about
to die. I felt sad about that, because my life
had been so brief, but I felt inclined to
embrace death with courage and hope, as it
seemed to be inevitable at that point.

When I felt that I could not resist the urge to
inhale anymore, I prepared myself to
breathe in the water that I knew would
drown me. Just as I started to do that, the
Light enveloped me, Peace and Joyful Love
filled my world, I felt buoyed by warmth
and Perfect Harmony. There was a sense of
a powerful Presence, which welcomed me
with overwhelming joy and love. I was
enthralled, delighted beyond words, for
maybe a few moments. And then suddenly,
it was all gone, and the surface of the
"water" broke apart and fresh air came
down to me.

At the time when I first started having the
dreams, I didn't know that I had been born
cynanotic (blue from lack of oxygen) by
emergency cesarean section.

At that point in the dream, I would always
awaken, gasping, shaking and sweating.

The dream persisted at regular intervals,
about once per year until I was 27 when I
entered therapy and received validation

about the dream being a birth memory. At that same time, around 1982, I began to see the similarity between that dream and the NDE's that I was beginning to hear people talking about publically.

That recurrent dream stopped quite suddenly at that point, and I began to work with it consciously. One of the first things I came to realize was that the newly-born me was royally ANGRY about being born after having had the NDE. Until the NDE, I had been keen to be born, but after the NDE, all the eagerness, plans and zest I had had to live was gone. After the NDE, life seemed like a miserable second best, a chore rather than the Grand Adventure it had seemed to me before the NDE!

I still struggle with that at times. Many times and in many different ways, I have been given the opportunity to learn how to accept graciously being given what I was wanting, after I ceased to want it.

Maybe it is like the Buddhists say, "Desire is what causes suffering. Cease to desire, and you get Nirvanna." I think that may be true, that as long as we want anything in this life, we create the energy which keeps us here, because ALL of our wishes ARE fulfilled, ASAP.

Anyway, thanks again for doing your site.

DP

NDE in Dentist Chair

In May of 1978, I went to my family dentist
to have a couple teeth extracted. What
started out as a simple procedure, ended as
a life changing experience.

A few years earlier, I quit a good factory
job to go to Bible college with plans to
become a minister. The plans ended early
and I found myself without money or a job.
My wife was pregnant with our first child
and we were without health insurance. I
tried to get my old job back but the factory
was laying off and there were no other jobs
to be found. With limited options, I decided
to join the army. After two (2) years in the
army at the age of 23 and a father of 2
beautiful children, I was honorably
discharged.

By May of 1978, I was in my second job
since being discharged and my life was in
turmoil. My wife and I were separated and I
was filled with guilt over leaving my
children. At this point in my life, I had lost
all faith in God and had no real religious
beliefs.

Soon after starting that job, I went to a
dentist to have a couple teeth pulled. The

dentist's office was in a small house that
had been converted into an office. From
what I could see, the house only had a
waiting room and a couple of patient rooms.

I was a little nervous when I arrived at the
office. I never had any teeth pulled and I
had never been anesthetized with laughing
gas. The dental assistant took me into a
room and she told me to sit in this old green
dental chair. The chair looked like it was 50
years old. She loosened my clothes and
wrapped a cloth around my face as she tried
to assure me that everything was going to
be ok. She then declined the chair and
placed a mask over my nose. She told me to
take in deep breaths as she turned on the
gas. As I breathed in, I could feel my body
start to go numb and my eyes became very
heavy. I tried to keep my eyes open and stay
awake as long as possible. Finally, my eyes
just couldn't stay open any longer and they
slowly closed as I started to sink into heavy
sedation.

When the dentist came into the room, I was
still aware of what was going on around me.
Even though I could hear him talking to his
assistant, I couldn't open my eyes and I
couldn't feel anything he was doing. He
started joking with his assistant about her
boyfriend and their sex life, which I thought
that was inappropriate. I wondered what

they would think if they knew I could hear everything they were saying.

I felt the dentist open my mouth wide and put some kind of clamp inside to keep it open. I could tell he was giving me a couple of shots but it didn't hurt. He put some cotton or gauze in my mouth and I assumed it to absorb the blood after pulling my teeth. Then I felt him stick an instrument in my mouth and begin prying and pulling on the first tooth. I was aware of everything he was doing but it didn't hurt at all, thank God! I felt my head pulled up and down as he pried and twisted on the first tooth. Suddenly I heard a loud snap and the first tooth was out.

During the time he was working on the first tooth, I continued to sink deeper and deeper within myself. I don't remember the extraction of the second tooth and I vaguely remember the sequence of events after that.

I felt my jaw muscles begin to contract and I could hear a buzzing sound that vacillated with each contraction. I remember wondering why my jaws were contracting and what was causing the noise. I continued to drift, as I sank deeper and deeper. I thought my consciousness must have been way down in my chest because I could see a light far away and I thought I was looking

at the light coming into my eyes. I felt
myself rush toward the light and suddenly I
found myself in another room of the house.
I was in the corner of a room, looking down
at the dentist, his assistant and two other
couples as they sat there drinking and
laughing. They didn't seem to notice me as I
watched them. The room was a light beige
or light green with two couches, a chair and
two lamps. I could not understand why they
were drinking and socializing when they
had patients in the office.

The next thing I knew, I found myself
standing in front of this great, misty gray
wall. I looked all around and the wall was
the only thing I could see. On instinct I
guess, I stepped into and through the wall. It
felt like a cool, misty like veil as it slid past
my face from the tip of my nose to the back
of my ears. Once the veil slid off the back
of my ears, I was on the other side.

I was standing in the shadows and I could
see a light in the distance. The floor looked
like it was made of a polished tile because I
could see a soft reflection of the light. I also
saw people walking around in the shadows.
One man in particular was off to my right
and just seemed to be waiting there with no
apparent intent to go toward the light. He
was facing the wall and was watching me. It
seemed like he was waiting for someone

else to come through. I couldn't forget him
because he wore a hat that was popular back
in the late 1950s and early 1960s. Just like
the one my grandfather wore when he died
in 1963. I sensed others milling around but
everyone was in the shadows and I could
not make out any other details.

Someone took my left hand and said, "it's
all over, you're home, don't worry about
anything, it's all over, you're home." I didn't
recognize the person but I've always
thought it was a woman. She just kept
repeating that I was home and not to worry
about anything.

A feeling of extreme peace and joy came
over me as I began to realize I was home
again. I was where I belonged and I was not
interested in returning. Then my mind
cleared and finally I understood everything
I had ever wondered about. All the
mysteries of the world were right there in
my mind. Not that I asked about anything or
that she told me anything, I just
remembered! I just thought, "oh well, I just
forgot everything while I was there."

I turned and looked behind me and saw a
large circle and in that circle, were smaller
circles. However, the smaller circles did not
fill all the space inside the larger circle. I
later decided that was an indication there

would be more people in my life before I leave this earth. In the smaller circles were all the faces of all the people that had been in my life. I looked at each face in each circle and sensed a rush of emotions and experiences with each.

My friend kept telling me over and over not to worry about anything and that I was home. I looked around again and it was as though I was standing on the moon looking back down at the earth. I could see scattered white clouds covering the deep blue waters of earth. It was very beautiful and I felt very peaceful and happy.

However, around this time I realized I had wasted my time while I was here. I don't remember why I felt that way but it was a strong feeling. Even so, I was still glad to be home!

I have always been a very protective person when it comes to the ones I love, especially my children. But at this time, I wasn't concerned about anyone. I knew they were ok and they would all be with me soon. But soon didn't seem to be a time, just that I knew they were coming after their journey. Where ever I was, I was home and where I belonged.

I turned and started walking with my friend toward the light and toward my home. However, after only a few steps toward the light, I felt myself being sucked backwards, out of the hand of my friend and back through the wall. The next thing I knew, I woke up in the dentist chair, alone and confused. The dentist never said anything about what happened that day and I never asked. I knew something profound happened that day, but at that time I didn't know how profound!

Fifteen months after the experience, my wife and I divorced. We have always maintained a good relationship and worked together for the kids sake.

Since the experience, I've learned to appreciate every aspect of life and not to fear death. I have to admit I fear the process and the pain associated with death, but not death itself. Nothing from my prior religious beliefs could explain to me what I went through. A large portion of my life since that time has been spent searching. Searching for my purpose and to make sure I don't waste the rest of my life. I've always encouraged my kids have an open mind about God and life and to make sure that they don't let anyone tell them what to think.

The things that were important to me before
the experience were not so significant
anymore. I no longer cared about physical
possessions or the need to pretend to be
something that I wasn't. Now I think more
of who I am and how I could be helping
other people.

For years, I didn't share this experience with
anyone. I was afraid of what people would
think. Now I tell anyone who will listen! It
wasn't until five years after the experience
that I realized I had a near death experience.
I had no prior knowledge about near death
experiences, but after that I started
searching and reading. One evening in
1983, I watched a movie that was based on
a true story, titled "Resurrection."

The movie was about a woman who died
and came back to life to share what she
experienced. She was riding with her
husband on a winding road along the coast
of California when the car went out of
control and over a cliff. Her husband was
killed and she was critically injured. She
was taken to the hospital and pronounced
dead on the operating table for about 7
minutes. Then she suddenly started
breathing again and she was revived. The
movie portrayed her experience during that
7 minutes in great detail. As I sat and
watched her go through the tunnel and to

the other side, it was like reliving my own experience 5 years earlier. I was really excited! It was as though someone made a movie of what I saw and experienced.

Today, I work in a good job, earning a fair wage and I do help people in my job. But it's not the kind of help that I really want to provide. For a couple of years, I volunteered with hospice. I talked to patients, family members or anyone else who would listen to what I experienced. I knew where the patients are going and I wanted to help ease their fears as well as those of the families.

My future will continue to consist of searching. I am still an average person with the normal problems in everyday life and I'm not perfect by any means. However, I've been given one of the greatest gifts of life! To know there is life after this earth and nothing that happens here is ever as significant as we think. I know I have to take advantage of this extended opportunity to learn, grow, share and serve.

The greatest gift I have to offer is my knowledge and to share it with people who want to know about death.

M. M.

My Story

Now if you will kindly spend the time, here is part of my heart. A mere glimpse of my story. It may not be understood by you, and that's ok. Those unscathed by lifes sorrows, or living above human suffering will be lost. Life is not a bed of roses for all. Some must trudge through the peaks 'n valleys mostly alone for the large part. And that is another deeper story.

Here's Why!

The childhood part wasn't cool. At a young age I started using alcohol and drugs (same thing). I grew up to be something I told myself I would never be like. I developed into something full of hate and rage, with a using tolerence and dependency to match. With no religious or spiritual upbringing to speak of. My only safe places were in the woods or being on the river here. (Well, back then the water ways were half way clean compared to now.) I felt a real kin to nature until all feelings became unknown and repressed except for that anger and rage, the rest were put on. School was pure hell, I was terribly over weight and withdrawn. Teased by teacher and students alike. Bullied and struck/beat as such on a

daily basis. I finally just had to quit.
Damage done.

Military time was a mess. I just learned how
to drink anything with alcohol in it, and
found new drugs. Discharged.

Also, failed at my attempts to be the
peaceful Hippie type. To much Dr. Jekyl/
Mr. Hyde. Finally at this point I was a fully
functional addict. Now finally realizing I
had to be just as crazy and violent as the
rest of the world, so not to be harmed ever
again physically. I done a mighty fine job of
it. That was my claim to fame -- to out do,
out drink, out use, and act out of total
insanity and hate. Have ya seen those
movies about the crazy biker types? Well,
that was me to the max. Be the first to show
up to the party and the last to crawl to my
bike and leave. (sold the bike)

So for years I didn't see a totally straight
day. It was all fun I thought, "until", it
wasn't much fun anymore. People all
around me were dying, suffering and losing
it all. A socially environmental norm.

So life went on as it does for people like
me. I tried to quit but could not. As I was
told by most and even those "loving highly
educated pro's," "you're a lost cause, no

hope for you". Twelve step groups had
nothing to offer at the time because I was
not willing or open minded enough. Too
much of that God stuff. And me being a
faithful hater even of the word was not
about to listen, or try to. (ego, vanity) So
more pain and despair.

I was now in another time of more serious
suicide attempts. But now I was going to
take some folks with me. Some I thought
who were causing my pain. It was all going
to happen on an upcoming week-end back
in `89'. But God had other plans for me. It
wasn't going to happen. I found myself in
jail that Friday. Saturday morning I was
forcefully, yet gently acquainted with God.

I was a withdrawing mess, suicidal, full of
hate. Alone in the holding, or so I thought.
Then it happened. In short, the cell took on
a different light and color. There was a
sound and intense feeling of rushing water,
but it was not wet or physical, it was alive,
moving and with voice, "living water". This
gentle loving voice said it loved me and
called me by name. By this time I was
pressed back on the bunk and could not
move. Physical breathing became nil. These
waters intensified, at a seemingly high
vibrating rate penetrating every fiber of my
being. I found myself basking in this ocean
of love, still held in total awe of what was

happening to me. (there are no proper words to use here)

To the Point -- the message; "to love one another". That is what I am to tell people, especially Christians, and their leaders, also to government officials. But, again few to none will, or have the ability to listen. Who am I to them? Just another tithe, a vote, a number, etc. (It seems our leaders have their own agenda). He said to tell you to "make straight the path of the Lord", "there should be no divisions but to love one another". I am to tell you that he "is coming soon". That we have "all gone astray". I don't know anyone in Ireland, but he said to tell them "to seek peace, stop fighting". And that we are to be "specific in prayer".

There is much more but for the purpose of this I hope it will suffice. Now, several years later I am understanding more of why and what was said to me, or shown. I asked the Lord who do I follow? What church do I go to? He said "none teach the true gospel, but to love one another". Starting my new Christian walk, unaware of all this denomination stuff, I found myself caught up in all the hatred, various "cults", materialism, power mongers, contol freaks (like, we will help you "if" you believe this, or do that), the so called best or biggest, the celebrity manure, and all the rest of the typical arrogant, superficial stuff. Plus being told by so called preachers that God would not use such a person as myself for such a message. Don't know much do they? He can and will use anyone he desires.

So I think you see I'm definetly not into the mainstream, or have a head full of the herding instinct, just to please, or to fit in. I don't "fit" in. I'm not a good game player "now", so don't expect me to be one to play that kind of game. Status or no.

The Miracle

That being the new person I am now. There is no trying to explain it. Either you know God, (not in a box) or you don't. I walked out of that little cell a totally changed man in body, mind, spirit, and character. Remarkable personality changes had gone on there, some intense spiritual surgery. From atheist to firm believer, with no signs of any form of withdrawal. I was over-flowing with an intense true (agape) love for everything and everybody. I had to really contain myself, I just wanted to touch, hug, and kiss everything and tell them/it that I loved them/it so very very much.

I couldn't wait to tell my story. Well things sure didn't go the way I thought they would.

My very first encounter was with the "preacher" man that was going cell to cell. Wouldn't ya know he didn't believe in that stuff, and really acted strange and in a big hurry to get away from me. He left me in a sorely confused state of mind, it just didn't figure. And I'm supposed to "shout what happened to me from the roof tops"????

So again I had to learn the hard way. I didn't have a clue to all of this religious stuff, and all the divisions, the arrogance, bickering, and hate. All I really knew is what happened to me and I just had to isolate and feed my overwhelming compulsion to read the Bible, and whatever else spiritual I could lay my hands on. I was held in awe again to find the exact same words that I had heard in that cell laying there in black and white, some times in red, before me. And it was with new eyes I was seeing this. It wasn't the same stuff I had read a little about or tried to use to mess with peoples minds in recovery circles prior to this.

I was on this spiritual type high for about a year. But now again I couldn't find my way, no acceptance, no understanding, no support, no love. Atheistic counselors I had been seeing were of little help, and did more damage than good. The same for the so-called church Christian counselors, as well as other scientific/academic minded characters. (I'll be nice.) Now I've found a few sincere folks out there, regretfully not in my area of the country. My greatest help came from a Christian therapy center. Now don't get me wrong. There are some good, sincere and well meaning people here, and else where, but we just don't click. Plus after all, I'm only human too and have my character flaws. Not to mention all the various experiences on my Christian walk making it difficult to tolerate certain situations. And with my past, I'm not real keen on the idea of this "do this to fit in" control stuff and all that goes on, like being accountable: to who and what? Or, subservient and yielding "without question". Again, to who and what?

After hearing the holy voice of the "Living Waters", am I to obey men/women instead of God? Was Martin L. King wrong? No! He was there in my so-called "vision." And I used to be a very predjudiced white boy. He had his dream/vision, and that's one I'll buy, "now". I don't know why it is if you're not in a clique, in their status, their partner, in perfect agreement with "their" doctrine, then you/I will not be heard. We/I will be cursed, accused of being an accuser of the brethren, or a blasphemer. At the least ignored, or not made to feel welcome at all. The older folks and others set in their ways refuse examination on all levels, have created untold harm out of their perfection. (Don't make the mistake of being new and sit in the wrong pew either). Too many talk the talk, but can't or won't walk the walk. Preachers remain silent in the pulpit to please, and stroke. Oops, don't speak too hard, might upset a wolf. Introspection, and truth hurts. Pharisees may topple from their high pedestals. Folks may hear the truth through their own ears, realizing they have been lazy and dependent on another's truth. Yet, if one speaks of individual truth, and questions, we are treated and talked to about terribly. Am I to expect that to be Christian?

What's really horrible is that I do not have all that "healthy" support. I don't have much family, no-one to really talk too. You know someone that has been there, done that, or that can at least try to understand this bitter/sweet passion of mine. Someone that won't say "I can help but it will cost you $400.00 an hour". Or the ones according to thier religious beliefs say I am to remain silent, not utter a word about it. It has really been tough to find my path in this thing. If you can tolerate a little honesty. That's why I say I just do not fit in. Seemingly around here anyway. That's why I belong in this rainforest. Away from all the games and hate. Oh, and concrete!

Dating has been a thing of the past. Been searching for that elusive soulmate to no avail. And I am not that bad of a guy now at all. I have to look at what our culture is breeding too, as well as all the superficial stuff, and what is called successful. Success to me "now" is not celebrity status, high scale living, having the most toys, women, drugs. Nor is it in our levels of education, pop culture, and etc. "We have all gone astray". It's not all that trendy, cultural stuff. But in love and charity, true compassion.

Now don't think I'm a shining example of Christendom, or some Saint, I'm not. If I hit myself hard with a hammer I'm not jumping up and down, flopping around like a cat fish on the sand bank saying -- Thank Ya Jesus!! Nope, not yet. heh heh :) I'm human (God it feels great), I know what I do Know and Know what I don't. I'm open and willing to talk about the spiritual path with anyone.

This story may be used, but not for profit. Also, it is not intended to be twisted (as I have seen before) to suit any one particular dogma, or belief.

Some parting thoughts for you to consider. What if you had something like this happen to you? What and how do you really think you would react? Would you be awe struck, or be acting goofy like some claim? Think

you would be able to get a word in
edgewise if the Lord was talking to you?
Would you really walk away with a hate, or
disdain for others of his creation? Think
after that you could live above human
suffering, and ignore it? Think you could
just give a little money and feel content in
doing God's wishes? Not the giving of
yourself? Think you would be perfect all
the rest of your days here? I really think it's
time people take a good close look at things
beyond their comfort/convenient/fitting in
zone.

"LOVE ONE ANOTHER"
And really ask yourself minus other's
interpretations of it....What Would Jesus
"Really Do"

T.

Why was I Brought Back?

I would like to tell my story because I do not understand why it happened to me, and why I was brought back to experience more pain.

Don't get me wrong. I am happy I had the experience. It's just that I have had to experience so much pain so early in my life (until I was 10, I lived with my mentally ill mother, did not eat regularly, missed one year of school, and basically lived in her world of illusion with her).

When I was 14. I wrote in my diary every day that I wanted to go "home". I was living in an abusive situation (verbal, emotional) with my step-mother and father. I wanted to die, had stopped believing in God (but had been an incredibly spiritual child), and was playing around with drugs and alcohol. My grades were D's and F's.

One day at school during class I felt only slightly under the weather. I hated school, and thought that if I went to the nurse I might be able to get out of school that day. When the nurse took the thermometer out of my mouth she gasped and said I needed to go home immediately. I was sporting a fever of 104!! It was very strange, because I felt only slightly clammy. My stepmother picked me up, and I think the nurse told her that I should see a doctor right away. My stepmother disregarded this and dropped me off at home then went back to work.

I started to feel worse about then, and went to bed. What happened next is strange, but I know it happened and I will never forget it.

In a strange half sleep state (some may call delerium, I was definitely feeling feverish and ill by this time) I started hearing roaring sounds, like planes and engines flying close to our house right above me and all around. After a little while of this I did not notice that they were growing silent and at some point I felt myself being sucked into a pleasantly warm black tunnel. I was swirling, sinking down this tunnel. It felt like it dipped down, and then started coming back upwards. As I travelled upwards I began to notice light at the end, or it was just getting lighter, or something. Anyway, the tunnel became a memory and I found myself coming up through a stream of water (like I was being born into another world through this stream) I stepped into the shallow part and looked around. I was in a very beautiful place. All vibrant green, and loving and serene. (The only really strange thing was that in the water as I was rising there were parts of broken apart fish in the stream, and some blood, but it was not at all scary. I am a pisces, and that is the only connection I can find). Anyway, I remember being very, very compelled to get out of the stream and experience that forest, or garden or whatever it was. It gave me such a gorgeous feeling. I felt like I was home, and like the place loved me, or knew me. So I started to walk into it, but just as I was about to reach the grass at the edge of the stream, I was sucked backwards through the water, down the tunnel, and up into my bed where I woke with a start.

I sat up in my bed and found that I couldn't remember what had just happened to me. I knew it was not a dream, and I knew something extraordinary had just happened, but when I tried to recall any of it, it was as if I was watching someone quickly erasing a letter as I was trying to read it. I got glimpses, barely, but was having a very difficult time constructing a picture. I immediately reached by my bed for my diary and started writing down ANYTHING that I could remember. I do not know how, but somehow I restructured the events. It took a lot of work. I kind of feel like I was not supposed to remember it, and that there is more to my experience than I've been allowed to remember. For instance I feel like I heard someone say "no", but I do not have a memory of it. I have a feeling about it.

Anyway I had no fever and felt like a million bucks when I woke up. I felt peaceful, and full of serenity. I felt like I could no longer be hurt by my stepmother. I felt lovingly wiser than she. I told my father, who had been like a great spiritual mentor to me for years, about what happened, and I think it scared him. He passed it off.

I was frustrated a little, but mostly I was filled with so much love that it didn't bother me too much. Now I think my father believed me, and knew that I had been there, but couldn't tell me that because then he would have to admit that he and my stepmother had been neglectful and that I could have died in their care because I was not taken to a docter.

Anyway, my grades began to improve incredibly, I just kind of stopped doing the drugs, and drinking, and I was more peaceful inside than I had been for years. I was at peace by myself. I took walks by myself to think.

I started talking to my higher power again too. I took great care of myself. This well being was with me up until I was just about to start high school. In fact it was with me the very day before I was to have my first day of classes. I was 15 now, and still a virgin. My life looked so full of promise. I was more confident than I had ever been, and God gave that too me.

The night before the first day of school I was raped by my best friend's "boyfriend". He was 21. Two months later I dropped out of school, and this guy terrorized me, and stalked me for 3 years. I did not tell anyone. I blamed myself. It ruined me, and life got immediately bad again. Worse than ever, in fact. I developed phobia's of people, eating disorders, and severe depression. I could not reach out to anyone because I felt like I was worthless.

My life has never been as wonderful as that time when I was 14. It has since the rape, been only confusing and unreliable. I still believe in God, but I do not know why that happened to me just after he gave me that beautiful gift. I have distant memories of being beautiful on the inside, like I was shining like a light. I have not felt that way since. Does anyone have any wisdom for me? I'm sorry this was so long. I just want to get everything in so that someone may be able to understand and help me to do the same.

Thank you.
A.

Before Birth Communication

After several months of trying and failing to conceive a child my husband and I were finally successful. We were both so happy. Our dream had finally come true. Unfortunately that dream was short lived.

Friday, October 13, started out like any other day. I went to work, ran errands, and came home. But then I started to have cramps. I called the doctor and was told to relax, put my feet up, and drink water.

I went to bed early convinced all I need was rest. In the middle of the night a little boy appeared to me and somehow in my heart I knew this was my son. I was so happy to see him, he was a beautiful boy, but he looked so sad.

I asked him: "why are you sad, what's wrong?"

He told me that he was going to have to leave for awhile, that God had something very important for him to do. He promised that he would return someday. I was crying, begging him to stay, but he faded away.

I awoke with a start and felt pain like I had never felt before. I lost the baby within 30 minutes. Although it was difficult to lose this child, I felt at peace that he would keep his promise and return to me one day.

He, Anthony James, returned the following year on December 3, looking just like the child I saw previously. He is a true gift from God.

Becky

Shirley's NDE

It's four am. She's standing off to my left in
the quiet darkness of my bedroom. I'm not
startled by her presence. She's been here
many times. I call her my water angel. Her
beautiful figure emanates light and love.
Her tiny hands reach above her head as
water flows from a vessel yet she never
seems to get wet. She is standing there just
letting the water flow. Her appearance is
almost Oriental, although she could be
Tibetan, maybe Indian, or Mexican. I
cannot tell, nor do I know why she comes to
me. She has been with me since my heart
attack and near death experience in 1984. I
need to record everything that happened.
I'm afraid that if I commit it to just memory,
I will forget too much. It was so beautiful; I
don't want to forget any of it.

It's eight am and cold as heck outside. The
room seems to spin beneath my feet. I feel
so tired. How am I going to make it through
the day? I wonder while brushing my teeth.
I could have taken the day off to relax but
it's not my nature. I have been driving
myself full out since the divorce and I can't
stop now. I worry about what will happen to
me if I do slow down, I know that the
thoughts, the anger, the hate and the pain,

they'll all be back if I start babying myself. I need to work. I need to be busy. I need to earn money. If I let my guard down for one second, I could easily become a street woman, living from one dumpster to the next.

I bring my thoughts back to the present, quickly dress and gulp down a coffee with mom, we are sharing a house together, since we are both on our own. She a widow and I a divorcee with three grown children. Are you going to the office today? she asks. You don't look well. Yes mom but only for a few hours. I have a date with Ron tonight. We're going to visit his brother and wife. Maybe play some cards. My chest feels so sore. I am having trouble getting up from the chair. What's wrong? mom asks. Oh mom it's nothing. I must have pulled a muscle, my chest hurts. We'll take it easy, you're always on the go. Sure mom, see you later. I stayed longer at the office than I had planned to and Ronnie was waiting in the kitchen when I arrived home. Ronnie I thought, how patient you are, how concerned. I didn't want to love him. Been there, tried that. No more relationships and no more pain for me. Besides, he is a farmer and that's the last thing I need in my life a farmer working a full time job. I had other plans, I wanted to travel and be free and freedom to me meant a fat bank account.

God my chest and shoulder hurt. Maybe I should take a couple of Tylenol before we leave for Ron's brother's house I say to myself.

Ronnie, a nature lover, pokes along driving the back roads searching for deer, ducks, big trees, you name it, he loves to discover it. I find this trait in him annoying. I am a get to where you're going as quickly as possible, sit down and unwind. type of person. He is an unwind all the way there type. Despite myself, I enjoy the slow drive into the country. I only wish I could see the beauty that Ron sees as he stops to watch three deer feeding in a grove, a few feet from the tree line. Or when he noticed a huge maple tree with half of its leaves still remaining in November and I comment: Wonder why the wind hasn't blown them off the tree, it must be sheltered from the wind. It blows mostly from the East this time of year, Shirl. They're the bad storms, never trust an East wind and the farmer was right to this very day I still don't trust a storm coming from the East. It's late when we arrive, but the house is warm and inviting. Ron's brother and wife have been quietly watching t.v. but they promptly turn it off. Soon the laughter and warmth of this house have me feeling safe almost like I'm tucked in. I love being with these people to this very day. We begin a game of euchre

with me, the bad player, winning. I wish the
pain would ease up. Not only does my chest
hurt, but my arm feels riddled with pins and
needles.

Dear God, I'm on the floor, I can't get my
breath. I feel as though I've been kicked in
the chest. Blackness. We're on the way to
the hospital, more blackness we're at the
hospital and I'm being examined by a doctor
and starting to come around. I feel
nauseous, but the pain has eased off. The
doctor confirms my suspicions. I had, in his
opinion, pulled some chest muscles. He tells
me, go home and have a good night's rest.
You'll have a sore chest for a few days, but
not to worry about it. I feel relieved to know
that I'll be okay but I have trouble getting
off the gurney. My left side feels numb, and
I can't get a deep breath. I want to go home
I thought as Ron helped me into the car for
the drive back to his brother's house. I'd stay
there until I felt better and no way would he
accept no for and answer. I didn't feel much
like arguing anyway. Even though the pain
has eased off, I cannot get comfortable; I
want to turn over and just stretch out in bed,
but don't have the strength. Eventually, I do
fall into a deep sleep and feel no pain.

Ron walks into the bedroom with a hot
coffee and says, good morning sleepy head,
it's after ten, are you feeling any better?

You gave us quite a scare last night. Well Ron I do feel better, if you don't mind, I'll have this coffee in the kitchen. I can't get up, my whole left side is numb, Ron, what the heck is going on? Panic sets in as Ron races me towards the Kingston hospital. He is not taking me back to the smaller hospital that I had been treated at last night. He wants me to be seen by a specialist in a larger facility. The top guns are how he refers to the doctors in Kingston. These words are music to my ears. There is no waiting involved when we arrive at hospital. I am placed on a gurney and rushed off to a room so quickly that I feel dizzy watching the ceiling lights whiz by. The only thing I can truly recall about the hospital are hands and questions. Can you feel this prick here? Can you lift your leg? Now the other leg can you hear me? Are you in pain? I just need to sleep and sleep I did. I was surprised to discover that I had been in ICU for two days. The nurse is moving me to a semi-private room. I feel much better and can move both my arms and legs now. I'm going to be okay. I think about what Ron had said about top guns for doctors. I am so caught up in my thoughts that I do not notice Ron sitting by the window. He looked terrible. The man is exhausted. I don't think he has the strength to get up from the chair, as he approaches me, I see raw pain in his eyes. He stands

over my bed, this giant man, holding my
hand, begging, please Shirl, don't leave me,
please. I knew then that I never could. My
strength was diminishing and we decided
that he should go home and get some rest.
We had both had a busy weekend. It's four
am and I'm wide-awake.

The pain, Oh God the pain. I'll ring for the
nurse, maybe she can help. Blackness. Pain.
I'm being ripped apart, no air. The warmth.
I feel a soothing warmth from my head to
my toes. A gentle pop of release and then I
feel absolute freedom and it feels so natural.

I am above the bed about four feet. I see the
body lying on the bed. I'm not sure who it is
and go closer to it. I just hover there looking
at the red hair spread out across the pillow.
She is dead. The eyes are open and vacant.
She's dead and I feel so natural, so warm
and free from the coldness and pain of that
body. I can see myself from all direction,
the front, the back, the sides. I see things
about me that I never realized before. At
first, I didn't even know myself. Suddenly, a
man is standing beside me. He is wearing a
long gray robe with silver thread woven
throughout the fabric. There is a dark gray
braided belt tied about his waist. The belt is
not sewn to the fabric, nor is it tied tightly
enough to keep it up in place it's there,
hanging down. He's an older man and I

seem to somehow know him. I can feel he is
totally trust worthy and extremely spiritual.
He spoke to me, and tells me that he has
been with me throughout my entire life, I
am having trouble with this concept why
had I not seen him before. Suddenly I want
to see Ronnie and my children to tell them
goodbye. I no sooner think this then I feel
myself leaving the hospital. I can feel the
wind upon my face as I race head first,
horizontally to Ron's house. He is sleeping
and I can hear his gentle snore. I can feel
his breath upon my hand as I touch his
cheek goodbye. Have the strongest urge to
move on. The man in the gray robe is fading
away gradually into the distance. I'm alone.
I hear a rushing sound. It grows louder and
louder every part of me is vibrating. I am
above the hospital bed my dead body
beneath me about 20 inches. I can hear
music it's the sweetest music I have ever
heard it is from a chime. I can feel myself
being lifted up as though I was being
sucked into a giant vacuum hose the
blackness is total. I have never seen such
blackness. I feel myself moving forward
through a dark tunnel, My hands behind my
back, my face looking straight up, the speed
I'm moving is incredible. I sense that I
could have stayed in the tunnel if I had
chosen to, I can see people in the distance,
did not approach them. I cannot express the
warmth and love I felt while in the black

tunnel. I can see a speck of light in the distance. The kind of light you would see if you held a black box with a pin hole in it up to the sun. I want to reach the light and begin to travel even faster towards it. As I get closer to the light I can see the figure of a man standing in the light. When I get even closer, the light becomes brilliant it's even brighter than the sun. Nobody in human form could have looked into that light . . . as my eyes adjust I see a man and run toward him, the lights surrounding him is brilliant and bursting off into white lights for some distance. And then the glow from my body seems to be drawn into his and he holds his arms open and I race into them. My heart is beating so fast, I didn’t think I could survive this. The love is overwhelming, we just stood there together and I cried and cried. He is younger than I had thought him to be. Jesus is a young man with hazel eyes and is rather tall, he is quite thin, for a man this tall. I realized standing there in his arms that my life had a purpose, had a reason for existing on earth. His arms slowly opened and I step back looking into his face and he says, your death was premature. It's not your time. No words ever spoken hurt me more than these words did....

Questions were coming to my mind my thoughts raced a mile a minute. Why have I died? Why has my soul come to him and

not purgatory? Trying to piece together my
Catholic teachings, His light begins to fill
my mind and my questions are answered
even before I could ask them. We
communicated without moving our lips. All
knowledge seemed to flow into me. I
realized that the grave is not for the soul,
only the body. I needed to know more,
everything from beginning to the end. And
as he speaks I am able to grasp things
immediately. I learned that this earth is like
a shadow of the beauty of the spirit creation
sort of like a negative from a photo. I
learned that the earth is not our natural
home. We are here to learn and that he
made each of us a promise that he would
not intervene unless we wanted him to. He
granted us free will to choose our own
path.and that each soul has the capacity to
be filled with love and eternal energy. I will
never forget his humor, he is filled with
happiness and there is a softness in his
presence.

Now I want you to go with this young man.
What young man? I questioned. The one
standing right behind you child. As I turn
around standing there is my friend I know
him immediately he is my guide and has
been with me all of my life on earth. He is
wearing a gray robe with silver thread
woven into the fabric. The robe reaches
down to his feet and is very full. It appears

to be many sizes too large. There is a dark gray belt tied about the waist area but not sewn into place. This amuses me and I ask what's keeping the belt up? My guide laughed at my question and said that I was to follow him. He led me into a large room where a group of loving people began to gather around me to say goodbye. Suddenly my guide is gone and I'm standing before a crystal table shaped like a horse shoe, there are a group of men setting and they leaned together to consult one another. One of them spoke: you must now return. You have a mission to fulfill. No please I began to beg to please let me stay here. I began to ramble and beg even harder as the tears ran down my face. The men confer again. Would you like to see a review of your life? I step to my left for the review. It occurs in the place where I had been standing. My life appears before me in frames moving very fast. Not only do I experience my own life and emotions, but also what others around me are feeling. I experience their thoughts and feelings about me. There are times when things become clear to me. I see the disappointment I have caused others and I cringe. I understand all the suffering I have caused and I feel it. My whole body begins to tremble. I see my selfishness and my heart breaks, the shame is overwhelming. When the review ended and I finely looked up I saw the love the council had for me.

They were not judging me I was judging myself. They all took turns telling me I was judging myself too harshly. The love in that room cannot be described in human terms.

Suddenly I was back in the hospital room again with the covers thrown to the foot of the bed. Lying stretched out on the bed is my body. I stand there looking at it, looks cold and heavy, and right now I feel so fresh but realize I will soon be back inside of it. With a swishing sound my spirit is back inside, the body's weight and cold temperature is unbearable. I can feel myself jerking around in it as if I am being electrocuted. I can feel the pain of my body the choking for air. I hear a voice say hit her again and the doctor holding the paddles, places them upon my chest. I feel the current of electricity lift me off the bed. Don't, please no...I don't want to be here, don't please no. I shout with such anger. I was fighting with everything I had not to stay in that cold body. The pain is unbearable, can hear the doctors talking amongst themselves and giving instructions to a nurse. She's back, one of the doctors said. Yes I'm back I think and drift into a long sleep.

I awoke to a bright, sunny November morning. My eye catches a movement in the far corner of the room. As he approaches

me I realize it is my guide and he has come
to help me adjust to my return to this world.
He tells me not to be afraid his love shines
from his eyes as he tells me you will be
protected for the remainder of your life. The
journey continues. I want to talk briefly
about the missing years and to explain how
I have been afraid to speak of this
experience until four years ago. If anyone
had tried to explain an experience like mine
my response would have been their nuts,
things like that just don't happen, but, it did
happen and it happened to me. I'm so
delighted to know that others are coming
forth with their own near death experience.

Yes I did marry Ronnie and we bought a
hobby farm and hoped to live happily ever
after but my Lord had other plans. I awoke
one night five years ago and was told now
it's time to fulfill your mission. It was to
build a cabin and they will come. I have
done that and it's been wonderful people
from all walks of life come to see the angels
who appear visibly, reassuring each one of
us of their great love and support.

Shirley.

God's Gift

I had a near death experience shortly after
my eighteenth birthday. I had been the
victim of much abuse during the previous
two years, and unfortunately, I admit that I
turned to drugs.

I decided to try some heavy duty
tranquilizers one night with a peer. As soon
as the drug began to hit my system I knew
something was wrong. I attempted to vomit,
but my gag reflex was not working.
Breathing became a struggle and I began to
feel delirious, out of my mind, inhuman.

I remember leaving my body sometime
before I reached the hospital. I remember
feeling an enormous amount of love and
care from my surroundings, especially the
doctors and nurses who were attempting to
resuscitate me. I remember looking down at
my body and thinking what a lovely girl she
was, and light hearted, childlike concern
that she feel better.

I soon felt a flashback at that instant, all the
way to my very birth in that same hospital.
My life had flashed before my eyes in
reverse. It could have taken an instant but it
felt as though it had taken the same eighteen

plus years as it had the first time. I then became aware that the girl was me. I felt somewhat ashamed, but forgave myself for having taken drugs and for damaging my body like that.

I decided that I was going to die. I did not see a white light, but was surrounded by beauty of all forms. I heard the most beautiful music, it was unlike any orchestra or electrical creation that I have heard on earth. I felt as though I were watching the best movie I had ever seen, and that I was the star.

All of life's questions were being answered, and I remember laughing hysterically and asking myself, "Why couldn't I remember that?? I knew it all along!" I remember putting the movie on pause and calling for my great grandfather. Suddenly he appeared and welcomed me warmly, though he was very stern. He told me that I must go back. The choice was ultimately mine to make, but that my death was untimely, and that I would regret it. He showed me a shadow of my adult self. I liked the woman I saw, and suddenly felt a desire to become her.

Then I looked down at my flailing body and did not want to return. I had dug a deep hole for myself and it would take many years of sorrow and struggle to undue the damage I

had done. I wanted to stay, but I listened to
my grandpa. I went back. I remember
coming to, and I could still hear the
beautiful music. This was God's gift to me.
He rewarded me for accepting the challenge
with waking memories of heaven's music.

A.B.

Bad Car Wreck

I cannot believe I have never looked for a place like this on the net before. I am glad I found it today. I have read many of the posts on your permanent message board, and whether or not most of these are "really" NDEs or not (many doctors say there is no such thing anyway). I would say they still all come from the same place. Blessed be to all of us.

Here is my story. 22 years ago I was in a bad car wreck and came to as they were getting me out of the car. I heard voices saying how bad the wreck was, and I was in a lot of pain. I started to "go to sleep" when I heard a woman's voice, and being a "feminist", thought, alright a lady ambulance driver, and came back. That was the first time they said I was dead. There was not a woman ambulance driver either I found out.

I had a bad broken jaw and head injuries, and they would not give me any drugs as they had to be careful due to possible brain problems. I laid in the hospital for 2 days as they waited to operate. My head was so huge and gross that my little sister puked when she saw me.

Then they wheeled me into surgery. I was prepared, my head/face really hurt and I wanted that fixed. I had cracked ribs and the last thing I did before being put under was to make the docs promise to not put the tray on my chest when they were working on my face. They agreed. I got more than one to agree. It was a big point for me then. (I was young ok).

Then I went under and the next thing I knew was there was this terrible noise in my ear, and there was a lot of rushing around and panicking emotions. I looked around and there were all these people I did not recognize, doctors running around this person on the bed and they were so frightened-seeming. I wanted to comfort them and remember trying to pat them or tell them it was ok. Then I looked again and saw this person on the bed with a tray on their chest. Then somehow, I knew it was me. I was shocked, really they had promised!!

Then I was gone. It was a whoosh without me realizing it for that. I was just in a perfect place. I knew who I was originally, and how my life had worked just as I, in my original, brilliant, perfect self had known it would. I saw how I had seen all the possibilities, was shown all the past lives of those I was coming to in this life, I understood the PERFECTION of life, the absolute perfect love of me, and everyone.

My life review was less of a movie of this particular life, but of more than this one, more than just my own 20 years, and I was surrounded by LOVE, LIGHT, and PERFECTION. I knew who I, my original I, was, and saw how perfect it ALL was. The whole scheme of us.

My childhood was pretty miserable, I had suffered physical and emotional trauma, and yet from that moment forward didn't suffer it again. I mean it was not important. I had chosen all of that, knowing it was for a perfect reason that I could understand so perfectly.

Standing in the light, around others of such perfection, no one I recognized, (I hadn't lost any close relatives so maybe that is why...), but they were my closest best friends, wisest beyond all words. I could never fully express the perfection/wisdom of life from that view. Like the world I had known until then was at the other end of the wrong end of a telescope and did not matter anymore. It was just the way it was, and was working just right, as I had known it before. I had just forgotten that. I had never known family love, and yet at that time I loved myself and the world more than I could ever have felt before. Acceptance and love!!!! It was awesome. Aaaaahhhh-hhhhhsome.

Then I heard this terrible noise, the flat-lining wail of the monitor, and the doctors yelling, and boom I was hurting seriously bad. My poor face. I could not see as my eyes had goop in them or something, and when I heard my mom, I motioned for a notepad and started writing it all down. I remember them reading a phrase, me tearing off a page, and writing another. We went on like that and I was so happy. I didn't "hate" my mom or feel sorry for myself at all.

I told the doctors that I had seen the tray on my chest, and assumed that the strange looks on their faces were due to being afraid I would sue for them lying to me. I had never heard of a near death experience and in my rather fundamentalist religious upbringing, this is not what I had been told death brought, so I never even called it that.

I always used to say "I was declared dead twice" and leave it at that. My own husband, whom I married due to incredible circumstances afterwards, thought it was oxygen deficiency. So I didn't talk about it much. Except to my kids. I have always been careful not to make death seem too "great," but I wanted them to know God is always there, and we are perfect, and to strive to be "best" here where we can't always remember that.

I also suffered depression, angst, etc. I would never have chosen to come back and do not remember being given the choice. But still, I must have, and since finally talking about it now to a few, I am glad I had that experience.

I have never spent a moment in 22 years afraid to die, or asking if there was a God, or wondering if "this is all there is...". I am not a healer, or written books, started movements, or whatever I might/"should" have done. But I am me, have tried my best, and worship Him/Her, the All-That-Is, with every breath.

I am lucky. (I have no external scars on my face which considering the way I was mauled by the windshield is an amazing thing too). I am lucky, as we all are, who remember, either thru one way or another. I do not recommend drug usage, tempting death or whatever, but we are lucky to have these experiences.

Blessed be, to all. Anon

My Greatest and Worst Night

Ok, here goes nothing. The first thing I would like to make clear is that I make no claims to being a writer. I just hope I am given the skill to get through this and hopefully have the experience come across as clear as possible. The most reassuring aspect of this is that those who read this will have a basic understanding of what this experience was like and the difficulties of trying to put it into words. I hope that you will also understand the fear I am now feeling while putting this down for others to see for the first time. This narrative may seem to have no rhyme or reason; I am just "putting it to paper" as it comes.

I would like to make it very clear, in the year 1986, the year I turned 19 -- I was not a very good person. Saying that never seems to convey the full extent of the matter. I was lost. I have spent many years trying to make up for the harm that young man caused. Many years hiding what I was from others. I am not now able to go into details, nor do I wish to. I would hope that I would not have to. Just so long as I can get the point across, I was not a good person.

The night of my NDE was the greatest and worst of my life. I suffer from hypoglycemia, low blood sugar. The bad news is I have to eat many small meals all the time or face passing out or worst. The good news is I stay thin. During this period, I had fallen into unconsciousness three or four times because of not watching my diet. My lifestyle did not help things either. I really did not care. I did not care about many things.

On this night I did not just pass out, I fell into a diabetic coma, extreme low blood sugar -- and died. At least that is what my "escort" told me. No one found me; I have no outside verification. I always wished I had.

I found myself alone in a place with my escort. I find it interesting how I tried to give shape and sound to things that had none. My mind was constantly trying to make the place into a room, and my escort --- just an entity -- into a person with a voice. I was there forever. The next thing I learned after realizing my brain would attempt to put a physical aspect to everything, was that when you are no longer of the body, time has no concept. As a "human" I still find that one hard to grasp. Moreover, harder still to explain.

My escort was not happy to be there. I could feel it, I knew. I felt like an annoyance, this was just something he (you will find the defining gender for this entity will change) had to do. He just wanted to get it over with; he had better things to do. He did not like me. This was his job, this was just something he had to do. I knew all this in an instant and I was trapped there with him forever.

After an eternity, I could not take it any longer and asked where we were. He flatly told me I was dead. I figured I was in hell, being stuck in a room I could not get out of (I had tried) with someone who felt nothing but justifiable disdain for me for all of eternity -- was hell. He felt this and, in the most condescending manner, told me this was not hell. I thought if this is heaven this is a real disappointment (not the words I used at the time). Again he knew my thoughts and continuing to talk as if speaking to a child he told me this was not heaven either. This was just a temporary place, it was not my time, and it was my fault we were there. We would just wait here until it was time for me to go back. He was sent to watch over me until that time.

Well I was one happy camper. I was dead, which was nifty since it was not my time, and I was not in hell. All I had to do was wait until it was time to go back – cool, I could do that.

After another eternity, I got bored and my
escort was not the most fun person to be
around. Therefore, I began to complain.
How much longer were we going to be
here? To this, he answered -- a little while
(insert reminder that time has no concept
when out of body). After another eternity, I
continued to complain. This sucks, I had
seen movies about people who had died and
come back, they said they had more fun
than I was having. What was the point?
Why was I not doing the "out of body"
thing at least? That would be cool, cooler
than hanging out with this guy. To this he
answered – you're too human. What did that
mean? I am too human. Of course, I am
human. What does that have to do with it?
He answered that my sins grounded me,
kept me away from my full potential (this
was a universal truth, not meant just for
me). They held me down; each one was like
a brick in a wall I built between myself and
what I was meant to be. With them, I was
limited to stay in this room with him. At
least he was starting to warm up to me. He
seamed to enjoy "enlightening" me, as an
adult enjoys teaching a child.

I knew what I was told was true, I never felt
the need to question. The answers were just
truths, truths I felt I should have known.
Maybe I did know them once, but not then,
not the person I was then.

Ok, so what you're telling me is, I am just out of luck. I am just stuck here with you for "a little while".

"No," was the reply, you can do something about it. Now he was really warming up to me.

Seriously? What? What do I have to do?

Well, he said, you have to "pay for your sins".

What the heck does that mean, "pay for my sins"? What are you talking about?

You have to face what you have done wrong in your life, I was told, truly face it. Then you will no longer be grounded; you will no longer be "human" (he always used that term as if it were a cuss word).

Ok, I replied, what is the big deal. How bad a person could I have been? I am only nineteen and the first like twelve or thirteen years don't count, right. So what is the big deal? Let's do this.

Are you sure? He answered. You do not have to do this; it is not your time.

Yes I was sure; anything had to be better than "a little while longer" with this guy.

All right, he said, it is your choice.

I would like to interrupt my story for a moment. I hope you can get an idea of what kind of fool I was then by my dialogue with this entity.

So it began, the story of my life. It was like watching a movie, only better. Yes the old "life flashing before your eyes" routine. However, it only "flashed" up to a point then it stopped. I was almost three years old, I realized that if I took things away from my baby brother it would make him cry. I wanted to make him cry. Mommy and Daddy were spending too much time with him and less time with me. The memory of what I did is causing me to weep even now as I write this. I felt (and can still feel) the pain I caused my innocent baby brother. I could feel the love he had for me, that and the confusion he was feeling over what I was doing. He was just a baby and I was torturing him for my own pleasure. I had to face this.

As humans, we make excuses. Some might say a sibling taking a toy away from another is normal, not that big of a deal. I won't argue that. However, I know that I will have to one day again face the pain I have caused others.

I was not facing this wrong doing alone. My escort, who now seemed to be a perfect entity, clean and without sin, was with me. He also could see what I had done and that I was ashamed. Yet we were not alone, the sky was fill with an innumerable amount of beings, all pure, and all were witness to what I had chosen to do.

Now I feel as if I will run into trouble with this description. I can not put into words the shame, disgust, guilt, embarrassment, sorrow, or self-loathing I felt over what I had done. There are no words. I feel inept in trying to convey the experience. These are just words. Human words.

These feelings actually took on a physical form in the way of an ocean, with no boundaries and no end to its depths. An ocean of regret with me, in its center, treading water. Every ounce of my strength I used to keep my chin above its surface. I pleaded, and cried, but the knowledge of what I had done, what I had chosen to do, would not go away.

I thought for a moment that I had been tricked. My escort was not an angel but the devil himself and this was hell. It was not my time but he was getting a piece of me nonetheless. Or that it really was my time and I had just chosen my own hell.

However, as quickly as these thoughts entered my mind I knew they were not true. I was just making excuses not to have to face what I had done. Not to have to face it in the light of the perfect beings that were all around me. One might ask how long this had to go on. How long must I suffer this way for the "innocent" act of a child? The answer is an eternity (no concept of time). In addition, the act was not innocent; I knew what I was doing and chose to do so.

Then it ended. The water receded and the emotions left me. I had faced what I had done. The distrust, anger, and the loss of innocence in my baby brother I had caused. Then the tape started rolling again, I had chosen this, I could not make it stop. I will edit the rest of my life down by just making a few points. Every time the "tape" stopped, I went through the same ordeal. The tape stopped for thoughts as well as actions. I would hope you could see how the tape stopped more often, as I got older.

I made an excuse for an action (well he did this to me first) which was met with a tidal wave of negative emotions that swept me under. Only direct prayer to God brought the level back down to its now regular position of just below my chin.

This went on so long that I had forgotten
what happened to me (a human trait) and
made another excuse, which was met by the
same consequences.

I only had to face those things I had not
asked forgiveness for through true prayer in
life.

I still had to face those things I had asked
forgiveness for through false prayer. When
I was just going through the motions. This
went on so long (no time concept) that I
made a third excuse.

I know what hell is. It was the moment/
eternity after the tape of my life ended and I
believed it would start all over. For the next
moment/eternity, I was among the others.
My escort by my side, she no longer looked
on me with disdain, but with love, as did the
others. I would like to believe there was a
little more from my escort in the fact that
she knew I did not have to face what I did.
It was almost as if she was proud of me, a
mother's pride in a son.

I know what heaven is. It was there among
the others. Again, the human words of
peace, joy, and love fail miserable to
describe the essence of being. This is the
place I remember when I face doubts. The

place I would like to talk to others about, others who have been there.

I then found myself back in the room with my escort. The mood had definitely changed. She was now a loving, caring, and understanding mother figure. Not the disappointed father figure I had come to be familiar with.

You will forgive me if I again interrupt this narrative. I am drained, it is late, and there is still so much to tell. I can not believe I got this much out on paper, so to speak. I am not sure if it makes any sense to anyone except me. Forgive me, but I do not know if any of you will believe it. I am frightened, now that I have put just this much of myself "on display".

If your responses to what I have shared so far are negative I will end it here and go in peace with love to you all. If you can understand what I have gone through so far I will gladly continue to share it with you.

Yours, Me.

First, I would like to thank those of you who have commented on my NDE so far. I am still amazed that someone can actually understand what happened to me. I have

*only known one person who had an NDE,
he was not willing to talk about it, and I
was not comfortable to bring up my own.
With your patience, I would like to
continue.*

I found myself again in the room with my
escort, only now it was much more
pleasant. She was much more kind without
a hint of condescension. She seemed to be
waiting to see what I would do next, as a
parent watches a young child who has just
learned to walk and waits to see where they
will go first.

The idea of an out-of-body experience was
still on my mind and now I knew I could do
it. I left my body and hovered in the trailer I
was living in, it was quite the remarkable
experience. After just a few moments, it
became common place, as if I knew how to
do it all along. I registered a strange noise
and went to investigate, but I did this
already knowing what it was and what I
would find. Information was coming to me
very quickly.

Around the front of the house whose back
yard the trailer was located in I went. There
I found one of my friends standing on the
hood of another one of my friend's car with
a large rock, smashing in the windshield. I
"stood" there for a while watching him, I

knew why he was doing it. I felt his anger. I also knew he was wrong. He had based his choice to do this on misinformation; I knew how he thought. I could tap into all of his memories, and did. I not only saw his life through his eyes, I could also see it from a third parties perspective. I could see the truth to all the situations he had clouded up for himself, and I was sad. I was sad that his life was filled with pain over things that never happened as he remembered them. Things he had caused himself. His memories warped by arrogance, greed, envy, and all the other common human frailties. I believe I would have cried if I could, instead I just stayed with him and hoped I could help him when it was no longer my time.

I then realized I could go anywhere. Again, the information was coming to me quickly. Distance did not bind me. Anywhere in a thought, and all I met were open books. Their memories were mine and the outside perspective was there. I could see their lives through their eyes and the truth at the same time. I could see how human frailties ruin us and bring pain upon ourselves. I learned that, for the most part, we are all the same. Thinking we are so different from one another holds us apart. I also learned that humans get very boring very fast. I no longer had human desires; the want to be able to go anywhere and know what people are thinking is a human desire. It serves what end? It taught me that we are alike, but then the lesson was over.

I found myself back in the room with my companion. I pictured her with a knowing look on her loving face as she turned her head slightly to the side and said. Well? As if to say what did you think or what did you learn. I talked it over with her. How we were all the same, how we messed up our own lives through our thoughts and actions. How childish and small we really were. How disappointing we were, and the fact that now I could do what I had hoped for as a human, now that I could do it, the act no longer appealed to me. She just radiated a smile so full of love I could have just stayed with her forever. She knew -- she knew all these things as if they were self-evident. Her reaction to me when I first arrived now made sense in a way. I was so disappointed. I thought we were better than that. That we, as humans, had come farther. We no longer crucified people in the streets, but we still killed out of fear. We still thought the same.

After an eternity with her, I began to feel better, but still I wanted to know how much longer I was to be here. I could help others now. I had information; I could make the world a better place. She just smiled that smile and said, "a little while". I asked what else could I do, what else could I learn? She responded where would I like to go. However, her answer was not limited by time. I asked her what she meant by "where". If I could really travel back in time. This appealed to me, I could see if we were better than those that had come before us were. I would know that we were not the same as those who had killed so many and hated for so long. She told me yes, but with limits.

I could only see though a first person perspective. The eyes I would look out of could only be that of my fathers and his father and so on. I would only know and see what they had. I agreed.

I could not believe I could find anything more disappointing than my fellow man until I took this trip. I bounced from one set of eyes to another, one mind to another. All were again the same. Hate prejudice, fear, greed, etc. They were all there and had always been there. I quickly returned to my room and again talked over these events with my escort.

How can the Big Guy put up with us? I am pissed off at us and I am one of them. How can God, who gave us the gift of life and free will, stand the sight of what we have

done with it? Her answer Â- Love. Well
how the heck could I argue that one, I knew
she was telling the truth. Love, and all that
comes with it, patience, understanding,
caring, and compassion. All these in a never
ending supply.

I had hoped we were better than we were. I
had hoped we had come farther than we
had. These things took time to get over.
After another eternity, I asked if there was
nothing else to learn, maybe something
positive I could take with me. She again
asked me where I wanted to go. Again,
there was timelessness about it. I asked if I
could see the future. She answered, yes, but
with limits.

*I would again like to interrupt my story. I
am tired and these pages just keep getting
longer. I hope you are still able to
understand what happened to me. I feel as if
you will and that gives me comfort.*

Love to you all, Me.

*I appreciate all the patience that you have
shown me as I attempt to tell this story.
Sometimes I am in turmoil whether to finish
the telling or to just quit and pretend this
has never happened. I have often wished for
just that -- that this never happened, that I
could just go on with my life believing this*

My escort told me that there would be
limitations to seeing the future. I asked what
they would be. To this she replied, "You
can only see what is to occur in your life
time". I could watch it from one of two
perspectives, out through my eyes, in which
case I would live it from moment to
moment with myself. Knowing what my
future self knew and thought. Alternatively,
I could be outside myself, as if viewing a
movie. In this manor, I found I could run
ahead and see what was to become.

This double perspective may get a little
complicated so I will attempt to make it
clear. For the next three days I lived inside
my future self, I stayed, looking out my
eyes, caught up in the experience for 72
hours, and then I "flashed".

"Flashing" is just a word I will use to
describe the following. I left my future self
and watched from the outside. From this
perspective I was not only able to see what
was happening to me, but what would
happen for each choice I made. If I had the
choice to turn left, I could follow that
decision out to its finality. I could then go

120

back to that moment again and follow out the path leading to the right and see what was to become of me. I would then "flash" into my self at the moment of the decision and try to influence my future self to make the right choice. In addition, when I would "flash in" I was aware of my future self's personality, how I would change over the years, how I was going to think in the future. I was also aware of all that had transpired from a, now, first person perspective instead of the third person perspective I had from just watching. I will try to clarify more by using examples of what I saw.

As I said, for three days I lived inside myself. I have to admit I paid little attention to what was going on around me. The experience was overwhelming. But at the end of those three days an episode occurred which made me want to flash (I will go into this more once I finish this future segment). I flashed and I saw the choices I would be faced with and the end results. Know this, each choice was met with more choices and so on and so on. The mind boggles at the amount of decisions we make in a day and how they truly affect our lives, the lives of those around us, and our souls.

When I witnessed a significant event in my life I would run it out, run out the other choices that I could have made, flash in and influence my decision. I was not always successful. We have free will no matter what the circumstances. I also want to make it clear that sometimes none of my choices had a happy ending, sometimes I had to pick the lesser of two evils.

I would then flash out and continue flashing in and out as needed. I quickly found out these few things. I would have to flash less often as time went on, fewer nudges were needed to keep me on course. In addition, for the most part, my decision to intervene was based on the perspective of a spirit being; i.e. I did not give myself lottery numbers.

There was at least one exception to that rule, something I did for selfish reasons. When you do something for reasons like that, you are going to pay for it. Every decision has its consequences.

Therefore, I continued flashing. The most surprising aspect I began to encounter was how the future me thought, so unlike the nineteen-year-old boy who was flashing. I was confused but proud at what was going to be important to me in the future. It was strange sharing the body with the future me, for the short period of time I chose to stay, before flashing. At some point my escort began telling me my time was short, that "little while" was just about up. I began skipping over larger and larger spans of time in an attempt to give myself help in the far future. Then, all at once I awoke.

My first thoughts were these. I am not going to marry my fiancÃ©e. I was giggling at the career choice I was going to make. I knew whom I was going to marry. Finally, I cried tears of joy at the memories of my children.

My post NDE life quickly slid downhill. Knowing everything that was going to happen for the next three days was hell. It sounds nice, but what is the point of living if you know what is to become. Worse still, I still knew what everyone was thinking and why, a gift. Some of you may be able to understand this one -- the thoughts of others will drive you insane. So imagine this, you know what's going to happen, you know what people are thinking, you know why they think the way they do, you know everything they have ever done in their entire lives Â- mostly bad, and no one will believe you and no one understands.

How long would it take before you lost it? Three days. I remember praying that night, I now knew that God heard all prayers. I cried and I prayed for Him to take me or to take the gift, I could not live with it any longer. And who to my joyous surprise came to me -- but my escort.

She was a ray of warmth, all smiles and love, and she asked me what I wanted. I told her to take it from me I could not bare it any longer. My only other choice to make it leave me, was to sin, and knowing what I did I could not bring myself to do that. (That might take some explaining).

She just smiled that knowing smile and asked me if I was sure. Something in the way she did that made me stop and think -- I then knew it did not have to be all or nothing. Therefore, we worked out a deal. I do not know how else to put it, and I am not yet allowed to remember it, but it has something to do with only receiving the gift as I can handle it. No, it has not been all peaches and cream, there is a passage in the Good Book that states the Lord will not give you more than He knows you can handle, and not what you think you can handle.

Well, I awoke not remembering. I knew something had happened but when I tried to recall it, I would break out in terror sweats. So it went for awhile. A few days later, I suddenly got the feeling that someone Â-me – was inside my head with me, trying to tell me something, and then was gone. This continued over the next few years of my life with the spans between flashes usually growing farther apart. Each time it would happen I would be reminded that something important had happened to me, but I just could not recall -- at first.

My life got on track; I turned into a "lucky" person. No matter what bad decisions I made in life, I came out -- eventually-- smelling like a rose. Sometimes it almost seemed as if I knew what was going to happen. Through it all, the fear I felt at remembering that night diminished and slowly, the memories returned, and so did the gifts. I was lucky, for the most part they came slow and easy, giving me time to adapt, time to learn control, to teach myself control. By this time, I was not in a position in life to bring it up to anyone's attention. I was trying to erase that boy of nineteen, and to bring this up, would bring up him. In addition, the career path I had chosen did not lend itself to this kind of experience, it would not have gone over well. Therefore, I was left to deal with it on my own.

I grew, my life went on. I learned to live with my gifts and make them a part of my life eventually. To the point to where I almost feel "normal", with one major exception. Every so often, I find myself not alone, for a few moments, I am here with myself. The nineteen-year-old me, is with me, a constant reminder that what happened did happen. An occasional nudge to keep me moving in the right direction. Some people find me over confident when they first meet me, they say I act as if I know the answers to everything. After awhile they say I am just "lucky" then, after more time passes, they just get use to it.

I know I am doing what I am suppose to be doing, my nineteen-year-old self reminds me. Every time he shows he brings a little more of that night with him and gives me a clue as to what is to come. He lets me know that what I am doing is the best that I can and he gives me the greatest of gifts -- confidence.

I am surprised by how much he and I have changed from each other, pleasantly surprised. Again, it is a reminder of what I was and what I hope to one day become.

I cannot put into this story all I have learned; I learn more every day. However, I would like to leave you with a few essential ideas if I may. There is a God and He will listen when you pray. You must believe He will never give you more than He knows you can handle (not what you think you can handle). Love, and what comes with it, will

get you through anything. Everything
happens for a reason. Finally -- tomorrow is
the first day of the rest of your life -- you
can start again.

Love to all, Me.

*(This Near Death Experience came in three
parts. I left the beginning and ending of
each part in because they are so interesting.
The writer is anonymous.)*

Meeting One

Hi Leroy: I read your article about near-death experience and I have to tell you that for the short space the answers were very precise and clear. I mean from my point of view.

My name is M.R.; I am from New York. My first language is Spanish. I will try my best to make my story the most understandable possible.

Almost nine years ago, I had I think was a NDE. Happens that I suffer from stuffing nose and dyspnea. Things that affect my breathing while sleeping. Well I remember that early morning, I awoke gasping for air but my nose was clog likewise was my throat. The sensation I felt was like having my trachea locked. No oxygen could get into my lungs. It was horrible; I still was half-asleep and began to extend my arms through the walls scratching them in intent of my body trying to find the way to breathe again. Was in vain, after all that struggling to avoid being taken for a force so powerful I was just remember being sucked by something as a huge vacuum that detached my life from my body. The experience is horrible when you are awake and dying by asphyxia you are weak but there is the feeling that you are losing your physical life. And then I knew I was taken by this enormous energy at a super velocity that I couldn't avoid, resist I was gone.

Then you feel going faster inside something that you cannot really explain with the adequate words. It is so fast that I cannot say it was a tunnel, I just can say that you in whatever existence you are transformed, this force takes you with such power that you only feel the sensation that you are going to a force that is claiming you. Yes you belong to it. I call it One. Then you know that you have left your body because once you are out of it. I saw down at my body and could see how my arms were stiff with the last movements I made while gasping for air. I couldn't understand how I was capable of seeing me and at the same time continue being taken by this force. Then I or whatever is you when you do not have body but seem to be existing in another plane. I was like in other dimension where everything was obscure. Then I heard a voice that I cannot say if it was a voice from a man or a woman, but was a peaceful one and told me; "do not be afraid".

At that moment I did not see anything, no one, any light. I just felt in such a joyful state of peace, no weight, I was transformed from physical body to just sensations; happiness, an enormous feeling of peace and love. Suddenly my sense of me went to another level, this time I saw that big or huge white mass and while getting closer to enter into it I began to feel that inexplicable sensation of being bathed in a beautiful warm and lovely light. You are just drawn to that irresistible mass of love. For me it was my contact with that Higher Divinity. I felt so good, so light, suddenly realized that I was free, surrounded by the most beautiful source of love. I couldn't believe that at the same time I was wondering how could I be conscious of what was happening if I am supposed to be dead. And I was getting closer to that white mass, suddenly my living force was sent back to my body. It was a small amount of oxygen getting back inside my body through one of nostrils that was slightly open. Then when the life force entered my body, I screamed "Padre", in English "Father". At that time I started coughing and my body was cold and shaking.

My niece who was in the bathroom when heard me screaming "Padre" so loud and coughing, she went to my room to see what was happening to me. I could hardly speak to her. I continue coughing and crying.

I told her, "G. I think that I died". She hugged me and look at me in astonishment. She gave me some water to clear my throat. When I felt calmer and the temperature of my body become normal; I explained to her still crying what I felt happened to me. She was afraid because in my face was the expression of someone that has gone through an unexplainable experience. She embraced me and cried with me.

Well since then my life changed completely. You are suddenly lit up from inside, and this illumination makes you more aware in how to understand what real love is, how deep we can go in trying to understand what death really means. How we must find why are we were returned to the physical dimension. Now I do not fear death or the fact that we have to go to other planes of existence. And I agreed with you in saying that you live with the sensation that someone is with you in the form of thoughts. I call that presence One. Because from that experience I learned that all humans are One connected to the principal One the "High Divinity or Higher Force". Sometimes I feel alone because many people say that I am crazy when I tell them my story. Others find it interesting and believe that maybe after all NDE is happening.

My way of thinking is every day evolving from knowledge to wisdom. There is a mind hungry all the time trying to understand things that before I wasn't aware of. I have the feeling that when I returned from that dimension called death something else entered into my body. And this thing guides me and teaches me by challenging my old way of understanding life, explaining me about how we can continue in the learning of what dimension is the real one or how both are complemented. I was always wondering how can a world like this continue existing with all that unfairness, humans divided due to continue stuck in their ancient beliefs. I was always vulnerable to the pain of the world, to its ignorance at all levels. Factors that I consider the culprits among others who continue being an obstacle for Planet Earth to evolve with the guide of One or the Higher Force. When I see people suffering or that I know that they are sick. I can't control asking "Are you in pain? Do you feel sick"? And there is the desire in me to embrace the person and transmit my love to them. Or I feel if I can just reach some part of their body or something that is close to them I can send positive vibrations of love that will ease their pain, illness or sadness. I can go on and on with the changes I continue seeing in my life. But at some point I feel that I do not belong to this dimension, and feel alone. Because I think that I am already dead or that I without wanting for it was taken to one of the most debatable mystery of life entering the other dimension where we are thoughts and emotions.

I receive so much data from "One" my companion from the other dimension that I feel like a torrent of energy greater that the capacity of my small body to handle. I sense that the High Force is so close to me that I begin to cry and then my body is drawn to a state of peace where I just fell asleep. For me it is like while I am in that state I am taken to places that later I cannot remember very well. Now I am more used to the presence of this Higher Force and I know when ONE sends for me. It requires too much discipline, practice to understand the changes in your life the way you begin to think. I wonder if we are living in an illusion or everything revolves around the mind; and there in the mind is the key to open The Pandora Box and finding the answer for the real truth.

For now I have to go. If you have read so far my story, thank you very much for allowing my soul to speak.

I wish I could contact those other beings who like me are out there watching and

bringing our humble light to illuminate
those who want to learn that this world
evolves and evolves without they having a
notion of how One makes the magic.

This site is so amazing covering all those
questions, doubts with such domain that it
has helped me to put in words what I have
gone through and the logic in some answers
are very good!

Thanks. Continue giving us light to see
where wisdom is hide!

M.R.

Floating in Mid-Air

The first thing I remember was floating in mid-air. There were no ups or downs, lefts or rights. It was just space. Thin air. So I felt like, if I fall, will I die? When I looked down all I could see was the infinite blackness under my feet. When I looked above, I saw the same thing. It was like a pitch black sky with no stars or planets or anything.

All I knew, I was somewhere very far away. So far away from Earth it was like a tiny speck of dust in a desert. I was beyond the universe somewhere where no human ever had been before and never will be. My thought patterns began to move slow. In real life, thoughts are rapid and quick, and come to you in an instant, but it wasn't like that. It was like someone put a TV on in super-slow motion.

If I was in the state I'm in now, I would have been roaming around and staring and trying to do things. But my thoughts became slow and unfocused like I was on heavy medication, like sedatives. But the thing that scared me the most was I lost all my memory right when I suddenly appeared in that blackness. I didn't know my parents,

I didn't even know basic math, I didn't know how to read, I didn't even know my own name. I was like some kind of undeveloped 5 week old that didn't know a thing about life. I just lost my memory at that very moment after I realized I was there.

It was the beginning of a new life. All of a sudden, I was "pushed" forward. I started to move so very fast, like in a blink of an eye. Faster than a car moves at its top speed, only it seemed slow to me. The tunnel went on and on and on and lasted forever. It seemed like a few hours before I reached anywhere. I lost all feeling by then except love, happiness, peace, and any other positive feeling. Fear left me completely. I was no longer scared of anything because I forgot what the feeling was like, or did I even remember what it was called? After that sadness left me, anger, pity, jealousy, and finally hatred. I was so different that if the person I hated the most was standing right in front of me I probably would have given her a big hug and told her that I loved her.

After a while, suddenly I stopped. I saw a blue light at the very end of the tunnel. I wasn't at the end though. The cycle was interrupted all of a sudden. But you see, that wasn't supposed to happen. I was supposed to reach the end and reunite with God.

I lost myself, but all of a sudden the memories and my ego have came back, but it happened so fast I didn't have any time to react. I heard a voice that went through every fibre of my body. It echoed throughout the whole universe. It had no feminine or masculine quality, it was just God. And I didn't need any proof, you just KNEW.

He said, "IT ISN'T YOUR TIME YET." There was no emphasis, no strange accent, it was just God's perfect voice. There was no way to describe it.

All of a sudden, I saw this bright, flashing white light. It filled up all the space. It wasn't blinding, because my "eyes" (I was a soul, so technically I was probably light too, but I couldn't see myself so...) weren't human eyes. I just saw. No other explanation. The white light was so bright that its impossible to describe. There were rims of perfect blue around him/her/it?? I like to refer to God as HIM, because that's how he describes himself in the bible... but of course, the human language really doesn't have much use when you're dead, because everything is so different. I can't remember anything after that. Everything went blank. I hope I'll remember what happened as time goes by.

All of a sudden, all I remember is staring at a woman. She looked young, maybe 18 or 19. She was my guardian angel, no questions about it. I was a human being again. At least somewhat. I wasn't acting as weird as I was before. I forgot the feelings I felt before. (In real life, I faintly remember them, but they're too incredible to describe.)

Before, I was innocent and perfect, but now I just felt like myself. Anyway, the girl was wearing a bright silky white gown. It covered her down past her feet. She also had two large feathery wings. She seemed like she knew so much more than I did, her eye's were exactly like Mary's. They were narrow and kind of sunken, but she looked really pretty. We were in a flower garden somewhere. She was probably picking flowers. When I woke up, I assumed I was in heaven, but I don't really know for sure. She outstretched her hand, but didn't say a word. I took her hand as she embraced me in a warm hug. Suddenly, I turned to look at a window that was taller than we were, and a balcony. I remember, when I took her hand, we traveled somewhere. Out into the far reaches of space and the stars. I can't even remember really. I think I was in my room.

Suddenly, I woke up. Or was revived as you could say it. I believe my angel was sent by

God to take me back to my body and come back to life. I breathed in a harsh breath of air. It felt weird. I looked at the clock which was 7:59 AM then suddenly turned 8:00 when I blinked.

My dad screamed "J, you're late! LATE! GET UP FOR SCHOOL!!" Strangely, I felt so calm. I got out of bed, stretched, and smiled. Usually I would be so mad and paranoid if I was late, but I was so relaxed. The whole day I was relaxed and happy for absolutely no reason. I was confused about it myself.

That's all of my NDE really. I can't remember the rest. It'll come to me in time I'm sure. I know God did say more to me. I just wish I could remember.

J.

The Oneness

In 1998 I was still in college, one day after finals I wanted to relax so I decided to go to a lake behind my apartment. I took a blanket, a book, and a bottle of water, and lay down by the water under a tree. I may have read a couple of pages but the birds were singing so loudly I couldn't concentrate. I was enjoying listening to them very much, so I decided to just look at the clear blue sky and listen to the birds sing.

My mind started to wonder how humans destroy this beautiful world, and wondered why we couldn't live with nature. I suddenly started to hear the most beautiful song I had ever heard. There were no instruments playing but the voice was not just a regular voice. It was so holy and very comforting. I started to be so absorbed in the song. From the sky, I saw a bright light. It was as if the light was a living thing. It was communicating with me, it asked me if I wanted to go to it, I did not speak, but I knew it read my mind. I wanted to go to it more than anything in this world, and then I heard my older sister's voice. My sister was pleading with me not to go. I did not see her, but I was telling her in my mind to shut

up and wondered why she couldn't
understand how good it would be for me to
go. She kept on crying and begging me not
to go. She told me she needed me.

It was my sister's cries that made me think
about this world. I started to think that I was
not ready to go. I thought that I was still
young and wanted to experience what life
had to offer. Most of all I felt my parents'
sorrow. At that point I was suddenly aware
of where I was. It was like waking up from
a dream, but I know I was not dreaming.

While it was happening, I was not scared at
all. I wanted to stay there and feel that
wonderful feeling forever. After the fact, I
started to get scared, to this day, I'm afraid
of looking at the sun. I still wear glasses and
close window blinds if the sun is too bright.
I don't understand why I'm scared now
because it was the most wonderful feeling I
have ever felt.

H.

A Miracle

On Oct. 16, 1970 I had a NDE. I was 14 at the time and playing in a tree when I came in contact with a 7200 volt transmission line. For 2 1/2 minutes I hung by the wire until it burnt through my fingers. I fell 40 feet to the ground. The kids that were in the tree with me said it was like I floated down out of the tree. They told me that I snaked through the limbs feet first without hitting a single one, and that when I cleared the last limb, it was like I stopped in mid air leveled out and hit the ground flat on my back. The doctors told me that that is what started my heart going again. What I remember is that as soon as I grabbed the wire, it felt like I was floating upwards. I don't remember a tunnel. But I sure remember that bright white light. It was so white, and so bright that I thought it would burn my eyes out. But it didn't, it felt so soothing, and peaceful in that light. If I would have had a choice I would have stayed.

I don't remember talking to anyone, but yet I know that I did. I can't explain it. I just know it happened. I was told that it was not my time, and that I had to go back. That I had a special purpose to fullfill and that when the time was right, it would be

revealed to me, (I'm still waiting). The next
thing I remember was laying on the road
and a motorcycle whizzing by my head, and
the neighbor lady calling to me if I was ok.

I passed out at this point. When I came to, I
was being loaded into an ambulance. My
dad had just got home from work, and was
able to ride along. On the way to the
hospital, there was the two attendants, my
dad and myself. But then I felt another
presence. I couldn't see it, I couldn't hear it
with my ears. But I heard it in my head. It
said, "Don't be afraid. Where you are going
you will be fine. Tell your father to take
care for your mother and brother".

I turned to my dad and said, "Dad take care
of Mom and Bob, where I'm going I'll be
fine". I didn't find out until many years
later, that after I had said that, my heart
stopped beating. They had to use the
paddles on me to get my heart going again.

After I got to the hospital, I was rushed into
surgery, where 3 doctors worked on me for
over 5 hours. When they finished, I was put
into a private room to die. The reason I
know this, is I came to and heard one of the
doctors telling my dad, "It will be a miracle
if your son makes it through the night". As
soon as he said that, I felt the same presence
that was in the ambulance. It told me,

"Don't be afraid. When your father comes
into the room, tell him you are going to
live". It no soon told me that, when my dad
walked into the room. I looked at him and
said, "Dad I'm going to make it". And I did.

Anon

Learn Patience

I had a heart attack, I went to another place.

It was like a room, but there were no walls
or floor. I was sitting down in a chair and I
had wings. There was a table in front of me,
and there were three men talking about me.
The one in the middle was the wise one,
you could feel his kindness and goodness.
The two on the side of him were upset with
me and were saying things about me. I
couldn't hear what they were saying, but
they sounded mad. I was sure they were
going to sent me to hell. To my left there
was a big stairway, going straight up
through the clouds. Thousands of people
were going up, I knew they were all dead,
they had no expression on their faces, they
just walked straight up. There was angels
flying over head. Kinda of a busy place.

I kept wondering were I was going. Finally
"The Wise One" in the middle, the one with
the beautiful white aura, came and sat next
to me. He started by telling me that I was a
lot better person than I thought I was. I was
so relieved. He told me I was going back,
because there was something that I have to

learn. I ask him what? He said that I had to
learn patience. Patience? I didn't
understand. He said it was very important
for me to learn this and he said he sent me a
teacher. I ask him who was my teacher and
he said John. John is my husband. I couldn't
believe this for he is layed back, it irritates
me.

I can't even try to describe the feeling of
complete peace, and everything is about
you, nobody else. It's a feeling I'll never
forget. I'll no longer fear death because it
was beautiful, no pain, no illness, no heart
attack pain.

Then I woke up with this chest pain, and
doctors and nurses massaging my body.
Asking me my name, and my date of birth. I
have since learned the meaning of patience,
and I hope I'm doing it right because the
other two men up there that didn't want me
to come back, are just waiting for me to
mess up.

F.P.

Sharing Love, Pain

In the winter of 1989 (I was 13), the filters that were on our furnace became clogged and carbon monoxide from the natural gas began leaking back into the house. I became very sick from the fumes because I stayed home from school "sick", but my brother and mother/father both kept going to work/school, so they did not get as sick as I did.

Anyway, doctors couldn't figure out what was wrong with me, and kept referring my mother to psychiatrists. We saw allergists during this time, and I was tested for food allergies (showed up to wheat and citrus and a few others), but this did not explain why I was sleeping 16-20 hours a day. Even at Christmas that year I was only able to sit with my family an hour before being too exhausted to stay awake any longer. These months were a dark, grey time where I remember very little except for this.

One night I awoke and found myself down the street, floating about 50 feet off the ground. I was standing upright, and it felt like there was a thin thread attached to the skin of my heart that was pulling me forward. I looked to my right and saw other people at different heights drifting forward in this same fashion. The direction I was going was eastward, toward a massive, beautiful mountain whose peak was obscured by a brilliant white/gold light. I had the impression that this mountain lay just beyond the edge of our world, not within it.

At this moment, I looked down and saw the road and Park beneath my feet and said to myself "I can't be flying" and suddenly I dropped from the sky into the snow. I looked up at the mountain again and thought "I can't get there if I can't fly." I was suddenly very concerned about not being able to reach the mountain. Then, I thought "hey, I was just flying, maybe if I re-create that feeling in my heart, I will be able to fly again." So I concentrated on my heart and focused, creating a sense of buoyancy. I rose up and moved toward the mountain again, much faster this time.

I came to rest about 100 feet from the summit, right on the edge of a cliff that faced the world. Soft green grass with tiny flowers grew here, and curled over the cliff edge a little. There was also a grove of trees loosely spaced around. If you can imagine the most perfect spring day, where the breeze is blowing and the world is waking up from a winters rest, growing. It was so beautiful that even thinking about it still brings me peace and happiness.

I looked up towards the summit and there seemed to be snow there, but emanating from the summit was this blinding white/ gold light. It did not hurt to look upon it, and it seemed to have form (light being solid -- hard to describe).

This light then pulsed at me, and the meaning pulsed through my whole being: "Do You Want To Stay Here?" I could not answer. I looked off the cliff edge back to earth. I could see the curvature of the earth, and clouds covering the landscape. I could see the individual street that my family lived on, and my house. If you were to look at a faraway hill, it would be like being able to see individual grains of sand and blades of grass.

I felt a concern for my parents, what they would feel like if I stayed here. I wasn't sure of what to decide, because I felt inadequate to make a decision. Suddenly, I rushed off the mountain and woke up in my bed, feeling so energized. The weakness in my body was still there, but it didn't seem as heavy anymore.

Within a few weeks, we saw another Allergist. She tested us for various kinds of chemicals. My Ethanol reaction was off the charts. She asked us if we had natural gas heating our home, my mother said yes, and the doctor said "you should get it checked."

We got home and called the heating and air guy and he came out. His comment "boy am I sure glad you called me, the filters on your furnace were so clogged, another couple of weeks and you would have been dead."

I took several years to digest the experience. The last ten or so, I have been living with severe environmental illness. I am so allergic to petroleum products and various chemicals (not to mention wood dust and indoor molds) that having a job or a home that does not have something in it that makes me sick has been an impossibility. There have only been a handful of days this decade where I felt "healthty" like I did before my sickness.

I am not afraid of death, I only fear to forget love/peace/beauty so much that it changes me away from being able to feel joy/ happiness/hope. It has been hard, my illness changes my moods to negative very often, but I have come to see these feelings as chemicals in my body, the "real" me is separate from my body.

It allows me to operate to a degree even
with severe pains shooting though my head
and other parts of my body. Soon I hope to
be able to build a home that will not make
me sick.

Sorry to ramble on like that, I hope there is
some information for someone in here.
Reading near death experiences has been
very good for my soul over the years.
Please do not be afraid to share yours if you
feel in your heart that the listener can
benefit from it.

M.R.

I Was Quite Ill

1988, I was quite ill, I lay down because I felt so weak. Then it happened!

Everything around me was getting dark and there was a very loud rushing of wind sound, similar to a plane preparing its engines to take the runway for flight. As it grew darker I noticed a jagged like opening that was so bright and I felt as though I was being drawn towards it at first very slowly, but the closer I got towards the opening I traveled faster, I remember seeing myself below, but the image quickly disappeared, the sound of speed was deafening the closer I got towards this tunnel like opening and I was curled up in a fetus like formation, I passed through and everything came to an immediate halt. It was silent!

As I raised my head, a wonderful and peaceful feeling overwhelmed me, I knew immediately that this was no dream, it was real. There were gentle rolling hills, flowers in every color, the sky a perfect blue, There was no one in sight but I could hear birds singing softly.

As I turned my head I seen a small cascade of natural white stone steps leading and

curving naturally to the top of a small
mountain, at the top of this mountain was a
large round boulder and from the other side
shone this incredible bright light.

I was drawn to it instantly, I began to climb
the stone steps, slowly I was in a long white
flowing garment and mist began to roll in
around my feet, a warm summer like breeze
swept past me, the strange thing was I felt it
pass through me and not around me, and it
was one of the most beautiful experiences. I
remember thinking to myself how is this
possible and why is this breeze making me
feel so wonderful, then came an answer, a
voice, "The breeze is cleansing your body
and your spirit." It was like someone was
answering my thoughts through telepathy.
All I had to do was have an enquiring
thought and along came the answer, it was
very comforting.

The intense feeling of peace is something I
don't think I will ever be able to put into
words, or even expect those who have never
had this experience to understand, but one
thing is for sure, I think about it everyday of
my life.

I stopped halfway up the mountain and
looked back at the beauty that surrounded
me. I smiled and kept on climbing, I had
never felt this good, this happy, or this

much at peace ever and at this stage I was
eager to reach the top, when I arrived at the
large boulder I put out my hand and touched
it and at that same time I did, things started
to go dark and I could hear crying and
people screaming, I actually heard my
family. I turned and looked back and I
could see them over my body, I was
saddened by the vision but I wanted to stay
where I was.

A loud male voice seemed to surround me
and said, "Jane you must return, there are
people who need you", of course I was
quick to reply that they would be just fine
without me and I insisted I stay, "Janene it
isn't your time and you must return" came
the voice again. The rushing of wind sound
started to grow louder again and the beauty
was engulfed by blackness. I held on to part
of the boulder as I felt my body being
vacuumed away from it. Then I opened my
eyes, the first thing I said was to my
mother, "mum oh my God am I alive".

Now people who read this may think I'm
insane, delusional etc., and of course I know
where their coming from because I would
of thought the same thing too. Before this
happened to me I was an atheist, science
was my religion, I believed when you die
that's it, nothing, there was no God, no
afterlife, heaven was just a poor excuse for

the human race to come to terms and cope
with the inability to accept death.

I was so wrong, there is life after death, and
the journey is like a birth of spiritualism of
one's soul and heart.

Jane

Experiencer Speaks Out

Hello.

I have had a lot of experiences and none of you seem bonkers to me.

I know there are psychics out there that act like they have a direct line to the here-after, and priests and scholars and politicians, but they can all suck on my big toe for just the least of what I have experienced.

And let me say this, it is one thing to be an angel and another thing to be an angel incarnate.

We hold the ball in center court and they know it. It takes no less than a great deal of bravery to pop in here.

Many, many things are possible. There are worlds beyond this world and there is life before and beyond this life. Much goes on behind the scenes, even amongst each other. We are not here by chance.

These are perilous times, there are far worse things yet to come. I am uncertain what to do or whether I should do anything at all.

No doubt there are great challenges and
opportunities ahead for each of us.

When you have lost yourself, and your
beliefs, and your fears; when you rise in the
morning with a heart full of joy, and lay
down at night with a heart broken for all of
humanity; then shall the cause of things
make themselves known to you.

Anon

*(This letter is a good example of what many
Near Death Experiencers feel. Tired of
being laughed at, frustrated with the way
people treat each other, but still absolutely
certain of their experience. Perhaps better
times will come through their strength.)*

New Year's Eve NDE

New Year's Eve Day, 1987, I was in a rear
end collision which resulted in my NDE.

But first let me say that I was pulled up and
out of the body before the moment of
impact! While out of the body, I was just
floating around the scene, enjoying a new
perspective which can not be seen from our
earthly view. My life at the time was pretty
confining so I was really enjoying the new
found freedom!

Soon, I felt myself being pulled into what I
later came to realize was the tunnel. Still, I
was just happy go lucky enjoying the
experience. I somehow pushed against the
sides and knew that it was an area that had
"sides". Soon, I began to see a bright light
at the upward opening of this tunnel. As I
noticed this, I also saw some "sparks" of
that light floating down to meet me.

Then I came into an open area with no
bounds that was super bright. Still being the
curious artist that I am, I started looking
around and up. Above me I saw the most
beautiful opening. You could compare it to
overlapping clouds with an open area near
the edge. But the "clouds" were the most

brilliant white/blue. I now am amazed that I could look at it as my eyes are very sensitive to the light. At the opening the "clouds" were lined with the most beautiful color you can imagine. If I put a color to it, I would say that the trim around the opening was a silver/gold but darker, not as brilliant nor as transcendent/airy as the opening.

In the opening was my visual concept of the kindest, most God like, figure that I can muster. (A jovial monk.) He gazed at me for a moment and instantly we were together "standing" at an invisible beginning of the combined energy of All. I knew that He, and the energy knew, that I was there and I felt the most complete Love possible. It was Love plus! I knew in an instant that all that I ever was and ever would be was known, not only known, but Loved and accepted. (I say Loved and accepted only that doesn't do it justice!)

This became a part of me instantly, and once it did my conceptualization of "God" directed me downward and to the left. There was a HUGE "Jesus" stepping out of some clouds. He faced me and there became a creation panel in front of Him. He was using what I now identify as laser beams, and within the creation panel were mathematical forms. I knew that this meant

that he was creating the events of the world
and my life.

Then I went down more through a forest
and came out near a cave. I think that the
"ladies" who took me through the forest
were my Grandmother and Aunt. Next to
the cave was my deceased Son. He directed
my attention into the cave and I could see a
wizard deep in the cave. I entered and I feel
that this cave was semi-circular down. It
came out on a landing, a dirt type landing
next to a river or body of water. The wizard
became an oarsman who pulled a boat up to
the bank and bid me enter.

As we neared the landing across the river, I
was told that I must go back! Believe me,
they knew what they were doing getting me
in the middle of stream to tell me that I had
to go back!!

By the time that we got to the shore, pulled
the canoe up and I was half-way up the
embankment, I turned around and said, "It
is going to be OK." Then I finished my
climb, made a right hand turn and awoke
strapped down in the X-Ray room of the
hospital.

I had not returned to my body enough to
feel that I was strapped down. I could only

see a green haze as my glasses were off. I only knew that I was alone and couldn't move and couldn't see anything! I bet that they heard my screams on the 3rd floor of the hospital.

S. D.

Wanted to Know the Truth

For many years, I practiced meditation.
With time the meditation became an
obsession, and every moment of my life
was devoted to it either directly (by sitting)
or indirectly (through meditation in action).
My sole purpose for living developed into a
limitless desire to know the truth about life
and death, to know my own immortal
nature.

During this time about two years ago, I was
teaching yoga and meditation to a cancer
patient, who was searching hard for
answers. I desperately wanted to assuage
his fears about dying and death, but did not
know the truth myself. During this time I
was forced to confront, head on, my own
fears and ignorance. My bones would
tremble, as I sat during meditation at the
precipice of life and death, breath
suspended for I don't know how long.

During these meditations there was this
infinite space into which I could never
venture. It was the "other side," and no
matter how much I consciously let go into
this space, I remained separate from it.

Then one day sitting on my couch at home, I began to settle in for a few quiet moments. When from out of nowhere, the infinite space that had always remained on the "other side," became the only reality I was aware of. It was like I was, prior to that, water trapped in a container, and then the container suddenly shattered and I was released into an infinite ocean, no longer able to distinguish myself from eternity, from God. No thoughts were possible, because there was no-one to have those thoughts, I was nothing, I was everything, I was what the words "unconditional love" point to. This was what I had been searching for all those years, and it was nothing like I imagined it would be. It was much, much more beautiful.

Then a little while later (probably a few seconds) and just as suddenly, I was returned to normal consciousness, where the "I" came back, and I was just sitting on the couch wonder struck. Everything around me was vaguely transparent and aglow, present as a reminder of the transient and illusory nature of the things of the world.

(The verbiage I am about to be guilty of is just my mind's way of trying to comprehend what was revealed. I have found out since that the mind is an utterly inadequate instrument for the task of describing such things, and it is good that it is so, for it confirms that God/Truth, is not confined to any one belief).

I had realized that I am not a conscious being walking this earth, instead I am conscious being itself, perfect and complete just as it is.

The experience of being a body and mind separate from all other existence was seen to be some form of divine inebriation designed to allow the show we call life to go on. If consciousness was not focused down into and through the individual, then life as we know it simply could not function. As someone before me has said, if we didn't have names and addresses, there would be nowhere to send the mail.

I have been reading a lot of people's wonderful accounts about their life-changing NDE's and OBE's. When a person leaves their body and sees that it is a bag of bones, and not in any way who they really are, the potential for fearless living is great. Through meditation and the grace of the divine I have seen that these bodies we lug around are no more us than a mote of dust on a distant planet. The only thing left to fear is fear itself, and our Real Selves are entirely free from all fear.

I have found that I have completely given
up trying to understand this grand mystery,
instead, I see that I am simply living the
mystery, living the knowledge, living the
love, as in fact we all are. I want to say that
it is possible to experience every moment as
a confirmation of one's inherently free
nature. And, truly speaking, since that
moment on the couch, I find it impossible to
experience anything other than God, warts
and all.

Ultimately I have no idea why I am sitting
here writing this today. But here I am, and
there you are. May we meet in infinite
silence, and sing together our journey as we
travel this incarnation of eternity called life.

Love and warm-fuzzies
Christian.

Pre-Birth Remembrance

Between my first and third birthdays, my yard included a special oak tree. We moved when I was three. Until then, my Oak was willing to be whatever I pretended it should be. After play, the Oak was a place to rest, providing shade on a summer's day. During those times, I first began my efforts to "see" where I had been before I came to this life.

I absolutely knew that I had been somewhere else before I got to this life. Back then, "seeing" where I had been had nothing to do with "remembering." With the most intense gaze possible, I would try to penetrate the open air, or an open area, to "see" the three beings who were with me just before I was born.

My efforts continued for years after we moved and eventually became a search to understand the experience.

From the beginning, curiosity was not my motivation. There was no feeling that "there" was better than "here." I was "here" on purpose. Those three beings were "where I was not supposed to be able to see."

Even so, I knew my three beings could see me sitting beneath the Oak. There was nothing frightening about that. That was the way things were supposed to be.

As I strained to see my three beings and their place through the open air, I was not seeking some celestial favor or gift. I was not seeking to return to where they were. The only feeling that I have ever associated with the place from which I came, and with the three beings, is an entirely unselfish, uncomplicated, and thoroughly complete love.

That Love was real at age 2 or 3. It exists as memory today. This must be the Love from which we came and to which we will return.

The remaining details are still crisp and sharp in my mind. That "somewhere" before this life was distinct enough to a "place", a special area, but vast enough to seem limitless. Light pervaded everywhere in pleasant pastels.

Many others were present. For me, only the three beings were important. They were there especially for me just before I was born into this life. They never treated me like an infant. I had no sense of being a "baby" during the time I was with them.

Standing in that "place" with my three beings, I was surrounded by spectacular vistas. If I had turned around, I would have seen the planet Earth beside and below us.

All of the vistas seemed unimportant. My three beings huddled about me, giving me both information and instructions. That was the important part. After that, they sent me here, -- to this life.

Years later, I watched three football coaches huddle with a player along the sideline. It was apparent that the three coaches each told the player something important about the game he was about to enter. There were instructions given. Then with a gentle shove, the coaches sent that player into the game. As I watched, I could recall my three "coaches" sending me here into this "game" in very much the same way.

Sixty-one years have now gone by. The Oak is as magnificent as an old Indian "treaty tree." A lifetime of experiences have revealed at least some of God's game plan for one man. Like all of us, I can not recall the information and instructions that I was given. Still, I have come to know that I am never out of His sight. No matter where I am, or when, His "still small voice" is a

constant Guide. Somehow my three beings
are His just as we all are.

W.W.

NDE Stopped the Abuse

Dear friends,
I had my NDE at age 8 or 9 during a near drowning accident at my local swimming pool. I had somehow got into difficulty, and found myself under the water, I grabbed a girl next to me by her bikini bottom, she kicked me away to the bottom of the pool, I was swallowing water fast. Then my life was flashing before my eyes, happy times mainly, birthdays, Christmastime with my family. Then I found myself in what appeared to be a large tunnel with a small white light at the other end, I was moving towards this light, fairly quickly.

Only my thoughts remained, I knew I was dead with a dreaded certainty, I thought there must have been some kind of mistake, as I was still thinking. I could feel an overwhelming sense of peace, surrounding me, enveloping me with the feeling, it was the most incredible feeling I have ever known.

As I was moving toward the light I could sense two other presences near to me, they were communicating to me through thought alone, telling me it was not my time I would have to go back. I knew these presences

knew me, but I did not know them, I had
never met them before, we communicated
just by thought, them to me, me to them.

Just as quickly as I had come, I was moving
back down the tunnel and into my physical
body, coughing and spluttering out water as
the lifeguard had given me the kiss of life. I
lost consciousness after and did not wake
up again until weeks later inside an oxygen
tent.

Before having my NDE, I had been abused
since the age of one and a half years, my
abuse had lasted right up until my NDE and
was set to continue afterwards. Up until my
NDE, my silence had been assured by the
threats and violence displayed by my
abusers, violent aggressive men, who did
not think twice about displaying violent
behaviour.

They had manipulated me into believing the
abuse was my own fault, and they made me
understand that there was nothing I could
do about it, by saying I would be sent away
to a bad girls home, by my parents for what
I had done, etc.

After my NDE I was so happy to be here, so
thankful to have been given the chance to
live my life, I really thought I was dead and
would not be returning to the life I had

known during my NDE. I could not stand
the thought of anyone hurting me again, so I
confronted my abusers, and told them if
they abused me again I would tell on them
and I didn't care if I got sent to a bad girls
home, figuring if I could cope with death
and come out alright, I could cope with
whatever happened to me because of it.

They agreed to stop abusing me, a surprise
for me at the time, I could not believe how
easy it had been, to get them to stop. They
realised I was serious, and obviously, they
could not risk getting caught so they agreed
not to abuse me anymore and they kept to
their word and left me alone. I still did not
tell on them, for fear of retaliation and the
dreaded bad girls home, but my abuse was
over, and I could lead a more normal life
afterwards.

I have blocked out all the abuse and have
been told this is called dissociative amnesia,
as I dissociated during the abuse to save my
sanity, though I was not aware of this, since
I was so small when it all started.

A doctor very kindly sent me a proof of
another person who had also had an NDE
and was abused as a child, though her NDE
occurred when she was an adult, which
helped her understand a bit better about the
abuse. I have never met any other person

who has had an NDE, and only recently
found any other places to do with NDE.

To die you'd think would be viewed as a
traumatic experience especially for a child,
but my NDE was one of the best
experiences of my life and the after effects
have proved invaluable in my life. I know I
will finally find people who can understand
what it is like through their own knowledge.
I did not speak much about my NDE when I
was a child, much the same way I did not
talk of my abuse, so I have not had much
communication with anyone concerning it.
Thanks for listening to my story.

*(Some further comments by the author of
the NDE.)*

That alone (the NDE) changed the course of
my whole life, I was no longer a victim, I
was now a survivor, and I've survived this
far, with only my experience to help me
cope with it all. I am so thankful I was
allowed to return and live my life, I have 3
beautiful children, who I love dearly and
happily, who have been brought up abuse
free, so I'm already making a difference in
their lives, by breaking the cycle of abuse.

I am grateful and never take anything for
granted, I help others less fortunate than
myself to get a better life, and speak up for

those that cannot find the voice or the self assurance to speak for themselves. I am an online volunteer for netaid and help in their important humanitarian issues, we can only hope and help as best we can.

My experience was one of the best experiences of my life, and will always remain a source of comfort when I find that life gets a bit tough. It really was the most wonderful experience of my terrible childhood, there for the first time in my life, I felt certain and sure, something I could never be, I felt loved and cherished, something I could never feel, and I felt valued and worthwhile, a thing I could never feel. The wonderful feeling of peace and love that surrounded me, enveloped me, is something I could never describe in mere words. Thank you for getting in touch and I hope my story helps anyone who needs it. Take Care

E.

Simile NDEs

(There are so many claims that NDEs can be caused by drugs, or brain stimulation, that the issue has become confused. I am including these simile experiences to indicate like-NDEs happen without any drugs or brain stimulation. Real NDEs, where clinical death occurs, can not be reproduced by drugs or brain stimulation. Knowledgeable NDE researchers agree, drugs or brain stimulation can not cause NDEs.)

I had an NDE (with a difference?) a fortnight ago, and since then have been scouring the Internet for info on anyone who has had a similar experience. I'm still shaken by it, and can do without anyone deriding it. Until it's happened to you, you might be skeptical, and I do appreciate that to some extent, but believe me I wouldn't go to the trouble of typing all this in if it wasn't genuine! I'm just hoping that maybe someone can draw a parallel -- or even just offer their opinion on what the experience is meant to signify. I've seen a few message boards, but thought I would post here first, although I don't know how widespread the newsgroup is.

By the way, I've never taken any mind-influencing substances of any description!

I'll try to condense it. I was asleep and suddenly felt a flashback of key events that had happened in my life, right from a very young age.

I remember "re-living" certain experiences (eg: starting school), even things I'd long forgotten. I remember feeling the same happiness, sadness, excitement, shock that I felt first time around. None of the incidents centered on family or relatives, strangely, but on how the events affected me (sporting achievements, receiving shocking news about certain things, moving home, etc.), thru adolesence, thru adulthood.

Then I was walking off a road near to where I live (nothing special about it -- don't know why that road) down into a bright valley. I was walking with a "faceless" woman at my side, who's presence felt just.... "right" (for want of a better word!) I started to feel the most unbelievable euphoria, happiness and contentment you cannot imagine. Honestly, it was totally indescribable.

The scenery was pleasant countryside, with a small village in the valley bottom, made of dozens of tiny hump-backed bridges and little houses and shops that looked "Dickensian" almost. My "guide" was leading me, hearing all my questions ("what's happening here? who are those people?" and so on) but always answering the same way -- that they had their business to do, I had mine, and I should not worry about them. They were pale, again, without faces I can picture, but bustling around and did not seem to be in distress or trouble. Yet nor did they seem to be as excited as me.

There was re-living of a couple of incidents which were intensely personal, and which I regret now, but I don't need to detail them here.

All of a sudden it was time to climb out of the valley with my guide, and though she was not touching me I nonethless felt many pairs of comforting arms around my back (though there was nobody there).

Comfort in addition to the supreme joy. I recall my saying over and over "I don't want to go yet. I want to stay here". Voices around me (not just from my guide) were saying "You have to go. Just be patient. Later. Later. Patience. One day".

I awoke suddenly, and for the next 30 seconds I could still feel the utter bliss and could hardly breathe, I was so happy. I was looking at my clock, evaluating what the time was and trying to work out if I should get up for work yet, but so happy that I didn't really care. Then the feeling faded in seconds and I caught my breath. The images were still right in my head though, (and the fact I can still picture certain aspects now, shows how strong they were).

No way did I think "That was a fantastic dream". Not for a second. It went far beyond a dream. The feeling had not been exciting in a sexual way or anything like that, just a feeling of "This is the whole point of existing", if that makes sense to anyone.

I had no-one at home to confide in, but after I'd managed to get dressed, I went around to my neighbor, still shaking. I could tell half of her thought "great dream", but later she started to open up and admit it must have been something out of the normal to get me in such a state. She is religious and wondered if I'd been given an insight into the afterlife -- and if so, I should be grateful, she said.

Re: my state of mind. I should mention that I had gone to bed as normal. I have not been

recently thinking about life and death, or
worrying about anything I assure you. I've
never feared death (but just want it to be
painless, when it comes!)

The voices saying it wasn't my time yet
made me think "NDE?" hence my frantic
research since. Nearly everyone else
mentions being near death (medically). I
wasn't. There was no "looking down on my
body". There was no "white light", yet my
guide had a glow around her. There was
absolutely no "tunnel". There were no
"relatives waiting to meet me". There was a
flashback sequence though, and there was
this joy unknown to everyone else, though,
and that's why I am treating this as much
more than a "dream".

My feelings now? More annoyance than
trepidation. It hasn't "proved" anything for
me about death. It's got me asking "What
am I supposed to deduce from this? God (or
whatever) shouldn't give me a sign of
anything unless it's obvious what it is!" And
anger that I want to feel that feeling again,
too soon! --Anon

Makes perfect sense to me. You had a
mystical experience, just like the ones
you've probably read about in the Bible. I

had one when I was 12- 14 and it changed
my life. For a long time, NDE's were the
only experience I could find that even
approached what I'd experienced. As I got
older, I eventually learned that I'd had a
mystical experience, which can be a lot like
a NDE, but not exactly the same. I also
learned that they're a lot more common than
you'd ever guess. Few people ever open up
and talk about them, so it's like the question
you hear kids ask when they hear the stories
about God and angels, visions and voices,
in the Bible -- which is why don't people
today have those experiences?

Well, they do. They just don't talk about it.
And because society doesn't accept that sort
of thing, they have no way to assimilate
them into their life. It confuses them more
than inspires them.

In any case, when I was young and terribly
unhappy (suicidal), I was lying on my bed
asking God for the millionth time why my
life was so painful. Suddenly the room
disappeared, and while I knew I was still
lying on my bed, my awareness was lifted
up and expanded until I not only could
experience all of existence, I became one
with it. To say that it was breath taking
would be a enormous understatement. Like
you, I knew during the experience that
"This is the whole point of existing".

The one thing that hit me so strongly
afterwards that I kept repeating it for days
was, "Everything is made out of Love,
because everything is made out of God, and
God "is" Love. But, if that's true, then why
is the world so devoid of Love?" I've spent
my life searching for the answer to that
question, and as Robert Frost said in "The
Road Less Taken," it's made all the
difference!

Later...

dg - "Keep an open mind, not a blank one."

Free Electron's NDE

Hello,

I found your site about 2 months ago, and I would first like to thank you so much for the help you gave me through your site.

I shall write down the best I can my experience and what followed it because maybe it could help others as others have helped me.

Shortly, to explain who I am: I'm a 48 old year woman from Belgium.

(I noticed that people from my country, which is very small, are very good visitors of your site. This amazed me first and then made me laugh! I think I know why. Belgians can laugh about themselves, auto-dÃ©rision in French.)

I'm French speaking, but have lived 9 years in the States while being a child. I had a Catholic education at school, but in my idea today, not so a good one. I closed my mind to religion and all learning of the knowledge of God the day I had tried to defend a 'black' classmate from racist attitudes of the professor, which was a religious person. My mother was called to come that day after school. I do not know what was told to her, but when she came back to the car, she told me angrily to close my mouth from then on.

My experience happened very simply, no accident, no illness, no drugs. But it's changing my life since 3 years now.

I was a part-time worker at that moment. My second husband was slowly coming out of big professional problems and my two sons, I had had with my first husband, were halfway to the end of their university study. This point was important for me. When they were young, their father had a very bad car accident and wasn't able to be a father anymore, if I may say so. I struggled for them. It was my main direction in life, even if I took some happiness for myself also.

Being home one sunny after-noon in spring, I just laid down on my bed with my faithful dog next to me. She was my 'mental helper' when times were rough. I wasn't tired, just very calm. Like a cat rolls himself around, nicely settled in a ray of sun behind a window. Sleeping in the afternoon isn't part of my habits.

I wasn't thinking about anything, just letting the 'black' of sleeping invade my mind. But, instead of falling asleep, the blackness teared apart and I was suddenly in a great light. I felt this immense love. A feeling I never felt on earth. No human love can give. Absolute Love.

I was I. And was with no more doubt or guilt of anything. A perfect state of myself, in perfect love. I was in greatness and I was greatness also. I didn't need to think to know where I was. I knew. I felt almighty. Powerful. I was pure energy. I was myself. And so much love around me, for me. And then I felt my love for my 2 boys and my dog. I said good-bye to them even though all 3 needed me on earth. I felt I could give them more love and help from up here.

I knew that my dog would probably suffer without me being near her, but I knew and 'told her' that I could give her something greater from up here. And she would also have a bit of this later on. I realized that I could leave earth peacefully. I didn't have to worry for her. I did not worry for my sons. They were humans and adult. What was up here was more important than my 'attachements' down there. But then, I realized that I couldn't stay there if I wanted them to succeed in their studies, they needed my working money. Right at that idea, I came back to my earthly-self, the light and immense love shut off. Only

leaving me a memory that something
happened.

I kept my eyes closed, trying to just get a
glimpse of that light again, even a small
point. I was sad, but not completely. I
scanned the feelings I had had. Trying to
get words on them and on that experience.
This wasn't in my knowledge. So, after 15
minutes, I got up, sat on the side of the bed,
patted the head of my dog and just knew
and felt safe for the 'after-death'. All the
other recordings just slid down and were
buried in my mind, not being capable of
understanding them.

I continued living as before, but certain
things didn't interest me anymore. It's only
today that I link these changes to this
experience. I let go of a lot of things. But
doing other things only for myself.
Somehow I became more selfish but more
self-constructing also.

Some few times I thought about what had
happened to me, thinking others would
consider me as crazy, though I knew and
was certain of something wonderful after
death. So, I shut my mouth as I was told
being a child.

Two years ago, when my husband gave me
a PC at home, I did search a bit on the web

about this 'white light', but not correctly.
Only fell on stupid sites. So I gave up.

Three months ago, I started searching again
on the web. In English this time. I read the
permanent board. First, I would read only
the NDE's that mainly spoke about that
immense love. I needed to feel it again
through other people's words. But I would
skip all sentences speaking of the Almighty,
God, heaven and so on. Not my stuff.

I was feeling pretty despaired. Things down
here seemed more and more ugly. Even the
sun didn't brighten up my days anymore.
One day, I was looking outside at the
landscape. The sun was shining nice, but for
me, all I saw was the black and white
impression in the eyes when the sun is too
strong. I saw all the bad done by humans
since the beginning under this sun. I was
thinking how beautiful and safe and soft the
other light was.

Then, I saw the limits of this landscape, this
world. It's hard to explain also. It was as if
the earth was in a big balloon and I saw it
blowing in, depressurizing. The blue sky
was waving like a blue cloth in a soft wind.
This world is finite and not infinite as told
at school. I was like having an electric
shower. In a fraction of a second, a sentence
came to my lips. God is all things. My

mouth fell opened wide. I knew. The
feelings here are also very hard to explain. I
felt the chaos of all things down here and
felt that up there, everything would be in its
place. More and more sentences heard in
the past came up to my mind. God is love.
We are God. All in one. One in all.

Ok, and then, what next? Jesus, yes, Jesus,
who is he again exactly, why did he come?
What did he say? I scrambled up the stairs
to my desk and computer. Thank God for
the web!

I was amazed! 2000 years ago, everything
was said about this. Why didn't anyone
shout it out louder? It's so evident!

Since then, I'm reading a lot. Trying to
catch up lost time. Also looking back to
what happened in my life, that's hard to
doâ€¦. I do feel being at a crossing point for
the moment. So, I just followed some tips
of your site and started looking around me
with other eyes. Changing my attitudes
towards others in small details. 24 hours in
a day isn't enough for me for the moment.
So much learning and thinking to do. This
does bother me because I'm neglecting my
daily obligations.

Oh! And I was very pleased to read in a
NDE that there's a sense of humour up

there. I like laughing and giggling. One night, I dreamt that I was a sort of tumbleweed having fun in the wind. Then next I became a sort of geometrical form, flying and rolling in this wind near the sea. Then I became a free electron, giggling and bouncing everywhere in the universe. Real fun!

This image helps me when I'm down and worried. A big smile comes to my face when I get this feeling of freedom again.

Since I haven't spoken about all this yet to my relatives, I'll just call myself: free electron.

Thanks again for all your work, you are helping a lot of people!

NDE on Navy Ship

During my time in the South Pacific, while in the Navy, I had a near death experience. Some of the details of where, when, and how, I would rather not go into. Instead I would rather focus on the actual experience because how it happened is a very complicated story.

Early on a Sunday afternoon I began to feel not well. It was kind of like you feel going into a bad cold or the flu and my stomach was upset too. We were actually in calm weather, with no waves at all so I knew it wasn't seasickness. I went up on the main deck to see if a breeze and fresh air would help. At the time I had no idea that I had unknowingly ingested a large quantity of a very poisonous material.

I went from being, not that bad, to extremely weak, couldn't move, my breathing and pulse were shutting down. My mind was still clear and I realized this was getting serious really quick. I couldn't do a thing but sit there and view an extremely beautiful bank of cumulus rain clouds billowing in the distance. Back-lit by the sun it was real impressive.

I began to realize if I couldn't breathe I was going to die and I couldn't. I began to experience some fear and anxiety, wondering about several things in a short time span related to dying and being alone when I did. That's when the real experience began to unfold. That giant cloud with all the shafts of sunlight streaming through began to have people and beings coming out, standing among the clouds, watching me and waiting for my death I presumed.

Had several hard jolts when I realized I knew them and they knew me. I knew they had come to take me up. After several hundred or maybe a thousand came up, there was movement toward me from the center of all the sunrays. As it got closer I could see there were more people, and someone sitting on a throne and his face was shining like the sun. I did notice the actual sun was still behind the clouds producing the sunrays through the clouds and much higher than the individual on the throne who was now very near the water, about 100 feet above it.

To get a better idea of what was going on, and what I saw, I would like to tell you some of the details I managed to pick out. I was sitting there thinking how odd. I really didn't have that much discomfort and no pain, but I was sure by this point I was dying, and these people had come to bail me out of a bad situation.

The whole time this had been unfolding our ship had been slowly moving toward the big cloud and seemed to have an accelerating effect on the unfolding of the events I experienced. I have to tell you some things about the ones that had come to greet me. Some, but not all, had angel's wings. About five of the ones with wings were fourteen feet tall! They weren't all together. They were scattered throughout the original group. There were another two that were about ten or twelve feet tall and looked a lot alike. They came with the individual on the throne. (Over the course of the next several years I probably ran into these two beings another two or three times. Apparently these two got assigned to keeping me out of more trouble.)

About a fourth to a third of the entire group was armed, and many had partial armor, no one seemed to have a full set of armor. All the arms were either spears or swords, some had medieval style shields. No one had clothing newer than the medeival period except one...my granddad. Up to the moment of seeing my grandfather I was being pretty calm inside. When I saw him I realized I would probably go with them. I knew what that meant. He had fallen dead

at my feet of a heart attack when I was 5
years old.

Also up to that moment, I believed
somewhere in the back of my mind I was
having some kind of hallucination, and I
would eventually come out of it. Now, I had
the realization that it was really happening.
I could still barely manage to blink or squint
and when I did the scene stayed continous.
It didn"t change like it would if it had been
my imagination.

At this point I really got scared, I'm
beginning to wonder who was this that I'm
getting so willing to give up my life and go
with.

The one on the throne turned to someone
off to his side, and that individual began to
make his way down the remaining clouds,
and walked down through the air to the
deck of the ship. This person was not too
tall, young, about my age, and built not real
heavy. When he took the step that put him
on the ship it felt like I, all of a sudden, had
several hundred pounds of weight on my
chest. I completely quit breathing and I
swear it seemed like the ship went down a
foot deeper in the water.

It was at that point someone alive, and at
the time, I thought a member of the crew,
came around the corner, said my name, and
asked if I thought I was going to make it. I
looked a glance at him and said "no, no, it
really was not looking too good for that". I
really don't know where I got the strength to
say that. But it was like a turning point. I
can only assume it was a blast of adrenaline
that pulled me out of this. The person the
one on the throne had sent, had only been
about 10 steps away and when I looked
back they all were gone.

I later realized the person that talked to me,
and unknowingly helped me pull out,
looked like a seven or so year older version
of the kid walking down the deck of the
ship. I also realized I didn't recognize that
guy. I thought I knew, at least by sight,
most of the 600 guys on the ship. I spent
some time trying to track him down to
maybe thank him, and out of curiosity.
Never did find him. Not the end, but all for
now. I later thought to look at the ships log
and see if anything unusual had been logged
that day and there were no entries out of the
ordinary.

My Near, Near Death Experience

For many months now, I have been trying to find answers on the web, answers to all the questions I have in mind after what happened to me 9 months ago. I came to this site by chance, and I feel some of you might help me.

Please forgive my poor English writing skills: I am a native French speaker.

I never had a NDE, properly speaking. I believe some religions call what I had: "enlightenment" or something like that. Sometimes I wishes it never happened to me, since I am now quite depressed. Let me tell you why but first, let me explain what happened to me. Last year, I had the opportunity to follow a 4 days training session: "From Alienation to Inner Freedom". To make a long story short, these 4 days changed my whole life. What I learned from the priest-teacher (a Christian Orthodox mystic) sounds pretty much like what I've read on this web site or other NDE sites...

A few weeks after my training session, I was reading about the economy, about the problems we all face today, about the fundamental macro-economic mistakes we have made during the past hundred years or so. All of a sudden, I understood all these mistakes came from one single "issue": we don't know who we are! We don't know where we are from, we don't want to know where we are going to, we hate to think about death and what comes after. We don't know much about our true nature and, worst of all, instead of trying to learn, we rather fight against nature, we fight our own nature. One symbol explains very well all this: the ouroboros -- the snake eating his own tail. This absurd inner fight of ours (eating our own tail) is the source of all "cycles" in history (the ouroboros is, among other things, the symbol of the repeating patterns). This is why, for instance, history always seems to repeat itself! But somehow, a tremendous joy filled my heart: I felt the "snake's meal" is almost over. An inner voice told me: "Don't be afraid! You see, 'evil' is just an illusion! Humanity is now getting prepared to break free from that illusion."

I also felt all the answers were in our hands, but we were constantly ignoring them. Why? Because we are afraid and we can't forgive! You might not see the logical link between the economy and our personal guilt and fears (i.e: what prevents us to Love), but this is a bit too long for me to explain on this forum. A whole book would probably be necessary. One day, who knows?

This is when things became interesting. Immediately after I realized all this, I began to FEEL a tremendous feeling of energy. I am not kidding: I felt Life, I felt Love all around! Physically I felt tremendous heat behind my head! It was exactly as if a HUGE fire was lit behind my brain but I never felt any kind of pain, quite the contrary. Sometimes, I had tears of joy, sometimes, I felt sorry and sad because I felt we were hurting God by our "ignorance of how much He Loves us". I also felt one with the Universe, I felt God was everything, everywhere. I could communicate with people without using words: I could guess what they wanted to ask me and they could guess what I wanted to tell them! Sometimes, people in the street came to me and started to speak, to let me know how difficult their lives were. I just listened patiently, sometimes wondering "why" they all seemed to trust me. Some people told me they had the impression they knew me. (deja vu?) I also felt for the first time that I didn't "HAVE TO MAKE CHOICES": all I had to do is to follow my intuition, so long as I was SYNCHRONIZED. Everything was making sense!

I could even guess where we all are heading to! Yes! I think I "received" some informations about the future, the way we are building it right now. We can change it, but we don't seem to be willing to change anything, unfortunately.

Words can hardly describe what I felt at that moment: I somehow knew "I was in paradise" or some place very close from it. I understood neither paradise, nor hell are "places you go to after you die": these are special states of mind, that's it! You can go to paradise right now if you want. I felt "death" was just similar to a "graduation party". "Life" is just like a school, something that has been granted to us for us to learn. Learn what? Learn to Love, which also means, learn to get back home, where our Father desperately waits for us. I know this sounds strange, but it is exactly what I personally understood at that moment. I swear this all came suddenly "from inside my heart", not from my readings! I never got that interested in NDEs or any paranormal experiences before: as an electrical engineer, I used to trust Sciences more than anything else.

My personal "inner visit to paradize" lasted about 3 weeks! Since day one, I knew this would not last forever, for I knew I still had many things to learn, many fears to overcome. I knew my "enlightment" was kind of a gift from God, to help me get rid of my Fear, my doubts and my ignorance. However, I never expected to feel as depressed as I am today.

How did I get so depressed? First of all, because it is over!!! I wished I never left that special state of mind... Perhaps you felt the same after your NDE, I don't know? I know I may go back there one day, but I am sometimes scared I won't...

You see, my sister, who just graduated as a psychologist (and she doesn't really believe in God if you see what I mean), immediately diagnosed severe "schizophrenia" as soon as I spoke with her about how I felt at that time. You have to know I somehow felt COMPELLED to tell everyone around about what I had "discovered", as if it was my mission on earth: Love people and tell them they should NOT be afraid of anything, no matter what happens! I also told them a few things about the "future" and this is where they all got really scared. My sister did a pretty good job of convincing everyone, including my girlfriend, my father, my friends, my brothers and sisters, that I was a "schizo".

My girlfriend urged me to seek medical help (she told she would leave me if I didn't). So I went to an expert psychiatrist, but he said I was OK and there was nothing particularly wrong! Unfortunately, this wasn't enough to convince anyone around me: they all believed I kinda tricked the expert. They believed I lied to him, or simply told him what I wanted to tell him. They all said they were very concerned about me, they were visibly terrified by what I've said. They all said they loved me very much and wanted to help me.

Nine months have passed since I left my "enlightenment" state of mind, and I still feel guilty for all the pain and the fear I have caused people around me. This new guilt I have makes me wonder if all this wasn't just a dream. Many doubts arose within my heart. Today, I am struggling with new fears: "am I crazy?", "does God really love me?", "If yes, why did he want me to leave paradise?"

I am wondering if all the ideas I've had at that special time truly were from God? Maybe my sister is right after all: maybe I appeared to have a mental condition because I accidentally let another spirit to take control of my mind? How else could I possibly explain the fear and the pain I have caused my family to feel? Sometimes they asked me if I became a prophet, but they were clearly joking. On the other hand, I have to tell you I really wondered at one time if I was not truly becoming a prophet.

Obviously, something went wrong and that something forced my friends and family to "reject" my experience, to treat me as I was insane. I don't know what exactly went wrong? The only thing I know is that I still can FEEL similar energy throughout my body for a few seconds when I am praying. This is the only evidence I kept to believe my "enlightment" wasn't just a "mental condition". However, I am scared to talk about all that today. I am scared and ashamed at the same time. Sometimes, my sister reminds me how much she feels concerned about me: obviously, she doesn't believe I am totally cured yet.

E.

Other readers answered E., so I enclosed their comments.

Hi E., welcome

You have come to the right place to post your experience. No, you are not crazy. Your friends just don't understand because they have not experienced what you did. It is not your fault they are afraid of what you saw.

What you did was normal, when I had my experience I wanted to shout it from the rooftops and tell everyone, but like you I soon discovered "everyone" did not want to hear what I experienced and became afraid of me. This is very common among near death experiencers.

So we learn to be careful who we talk to about our experience, and form support groups, and message boards such as this one.

It is also normal to feel "let down" after the passage of time, but there is much to do and many to help. Each of us, including you, have a mission on this earth. You may know what it is already, or you may learn as time goes by. It would be good for you to read and study the experiences of others. This will help you adjust to your new knowledge and show you ways of using it constructively to help others.

Just living an honest, truthful, and kind life will help ever so many to know that it is possible and desirable to do this.

Perhaps you will write your experience in a book, and/ or post it elsewhere so others can read it. What you do and become here on earth is your choice.

Jesus said: "Blessed are those that have not seen, yet believe."

When you become depressed, remember the greater whole of everything and how fortunate you are to have seen it. Know that it is yours forever, and no one can take it from you. The "energy" you still feel will remain to remind you. I still feel the energy after 16 years.

Love and God Bless. Choose only love. L.

Hi E.

For a French speaking person, you write very well in English! I'm also French speaking and I suppose that you, like me, didn't find anything serious on the web in French concerning nde. Apparently, in the French culture, ndes are immediately linked with turning tables, ufo's, and other types of sects. Don't forget, the French revolution abolished the catholic church and God with it. Ils ont jete le bebe avec l'eau de la baignoire !

I understand very well your problems with people surrounding you. I think that we'll have more difficulties to convince anyone in the French culture than in the English culture. But hold on to your truth! You see, just right now, you made someone happy: me. I know now I'm not alone across the ocean.

My opinion would be to stay free from all religions or sects, our families and friends are right on this point to fear for us.

I admire your courage to have gone to a psychiatrist when your family asked it! My brother-in-law is a neuro-psychiatrist and, just one time, I let out laughing, after a wedding mass, the sentence: 'No, I wasn't bathing in The Light during the mass'. He lifted up his eyebrow so high that I understood that even this was a step too far.

My husband, to whom I spoke of my experience one day he was having heart problems â€“ I thought that I could soften his fear of death -- got so upset that I could get involved with sects or churches (grenouille de benitier) that I gave up all conversations of God, life after life or anything else with him. But I stand up when justice isn't respected.

Our friend Lekatt is right to advise you to read all other ndes that you can. Even if this won't tell you what to do exactly in your particular life, it brings back that wonderful feeling of love.

Many of us are homesick. This is probably one of our trials on earth. Feeling ungifted after a while apparently is a normal process. Les secheresses de l'ame as the great French mystics write about it! Reading these old books helped me understand a lot of what was happening to me. Therese d'Avila and St. Jean de la Croix had hard times to explain and write what they experienced in those ancient times! You'll find them on the net in French.

My first son is a freshly graduated electronic engineer, I hope and pray that he too, and my second son also, may one day see the light!

Don't feel guilty if you got your friends and family upset, it will make them think a bit, be more aware of certain things, maybe later on. It wasn't useless.

Hold on and have a nice day exploring life on earth!

And once more, thanks to Lekatt for this forum!

(I hope that one day, there will be an honest one in French!)

G.

My Pre-Birth Experience

My boyfriend says it's impossible to have
memories before you have a brain, but I'm
here to tell him and anyone else who wants
to listen that there is life before you're born.

I remember being in heaven.

The whole place was lit up with a very
bright light, illuminating from everywhere.

I remember I was sitting on a white wooden
swing next to a woman who was to my
right. She seemed like a mother figure to
me, (but since when you're in heaven
everyone is connected, it could have just
been that.)

I remember looking down at my legs as we
where swinging gently and thinking I must
be about 5 years old. Although in my mind I
felt to be an adult and much more intelligent
that a 5 year old should be. As we sat
swinging I could see people sitting around
on the ground relaxing and talking happily.

There was a huge gate made of white shiny
swirled stone trimmed in gold straight
ahead and to my right. In front of the gate
there was a giant palm tree that was even

taller than the gate and quite big in circumference.

Leading up to the gate and in front of where I was sitting was a long gold path. The path was as smooth as glass with the depth of water on a calm day.

Also to the right hand side of the gold path there where people sitting on what looked to be the freshest baby green grass. There was about four of them. They where just relaxing like myself and the woman next to me.

Then I saw God, and he was wearing white robe. We all saw him walking down the gold path, and everyone turned to look, we knew he was coming to me.

Everyone was watching now, and I felt so proud. When he stopped to stand in front of me, he just looked at me and without words I knew I was going to be born.

It was a mutual understanding, all without a word being spoken. I felt as if this was the moment. I could feel everyone's excitement and I was ready.

Then I remember panicking and thinking to myself that I didn't want to forget heaven.

I knew where I was going to be (in the flesh) and I knew how easy it was to forget heaven while in the flesh, and I sat there trying to remember every moment. Looking around me and taking in what I could as quickly as I could, all while telling myself never to forget.

I felt that for me to forget heaven was shameful, how could I? It seemed impossible, but I knew many people did forget heaven and I wasn't going to let myself forget. Although I knew that's just the way it was supposed to be. I was planning to remember no matter what the cost. It was just SO IMPORTANT to me. All I could think was, it's real now but just like a dream I could see myself waking and wondering one day if what I saw was true. And it made me feel so bad inside knowing that is was possible to forget. I just couldn't allow myself, I couldn't.

Then I felt God looking proudly upon me, and I knew then that he would not let me forget heaven. I felt as though he believed he had made a good choice in sending me here. I felt as though he had something planned through me but I didn't know what it was although I know it was something he had given great thought to, and was happy with his choice in me. I plan to never let him down.

I know I may not have conveyed this
message of heaven as well as it was.

I don't believe anyone could do heaven
justice with mere words, but believe me
when I tell you it is real.

If you are alive and reading this now YOU
HAVE BEEN TO HEAVEN. You couldn't
be here otherwise. I know how easy it is to
forget, but it's such a wonderful fantastic
place.

I wish you could remember before you die.
I know after death you'll say to yourself. "It
is here!!" You'll feel so at one with the
world, life, and totally at peace. Everything
will make perfect sense and some of you
will wonder why you found it so hard to
believe in the first place.

Earth, and the flesh that once was will
become like the dream heaven is to you
now. You'll finally be home, and that
something you've always looked for will
finally be found.

Even if you don't believe me now, I KNOW
you will be there again some day and you
WILL BELIEVE. You'll wonder how you
could have ever forgotten.

BTW: I am willing to take a lie detector test
to prove all that I have stated above is the
truth to the best of my memory.

J.

The Light of God's Love

I prefer to remain anonymous about my experience. For reference, I send you my city and year of birth (see it at the end).

BRIEF DESCRIPTION OF MY NDE-LIKE OR STE:

The following is a brief description of my experience as I described it to a person in an e-mail:

Yes, I don't mind sharing my experience with you. It was a spontaneous NDE-like which happened to me when I was around 11 years old. I have written it down.

Let me briefly tell you a little bit about myself, about my experience, and about how I feel about this issue.

My experience happened to me in around 1974, when I was 11 years old (more or less). Now I am 40 years old (2004). In that time, I lived in a small town in the south of Spain, Montilla (Cordoba). One day I was sitting in class with my classmates and my teacher. It was a completely regular day, everything was going normally, I was in perfect condition, good health, etc. I was

watching how the teacher was preparing
something to show it to us, and waiting for
him to finish it, when, all of a sudden, I
started to feel and very clearly perceive that
something REALLY GOOD was
approaching the room from behind the right
hand wall.

I noticed that it was coming closer, and
closer. It had the feeling of intense,
wonderful, soft, nice and familiar TRUE
LOVE (somehow I had the feeling that I
knew that LOVE, but I couldn't tell you
how).

Gradually the room started to get full of
light. It was white light, it got stronger and
stronger.

I kept thinking all the time: "this is
wonderful...so, it really existed!" (I meant
God and those type of things, etc.)

I then found myself inside of this incredible
HUGE and VERY, VERY BRILLIANT
PURE WHITE LIGHT, although the center
of it seemed to be a little further away in
front of me.

The light was HUGE, coming from
everywhere, and it was POWERFUL
(stronger and bigger than the sun). It was

like a HUGE swimming pool full of light
instead of water (better yet, an ocean). I
mean that everywhere you looked, there
was white light, only white light. But the
light was beautiful to look at (I don't know
why), and it did not hurt my eyes.

I have spent the rest of my life looking at
very bright lights to compare them to that
light. (Example: tennis courts lights,
powerful lights that they use for video
cameras in weddings, the sun, etc.) But they
cannot compare AT ALL to that one, and
they do hurt my eyes.

Anyhow, I wanted to get closer to the center
of the light. At that point I was not aware
anymore of my surroundings in the class,
and when I tried to move closer to it, I felt
like a "strong pull" towards the center of the
light. Or maybe I made an effort to go in
that direction. I am not quite sure about that.
I was indeed VERY curious to get closer to
it, but I believe I was not in control of what
was happening or where I was going.

Anyhow, the LIGHT irradiated a VERY
HIGH DOSE OF PURE TRUE LOVE. I
could not explain to you how HIGH. I write
in capital letters because there are no words
in our vocabulary to describe it. The
intensity of it is not of this world!!!

Since then, I've learned there is nothing else in this world that could make us TOTALLY happy -- nothing!! Not money, expensive cars, earthly pleasures, etc., etc., unless it is similar to that light, and I haven't found yet anything like that LIGHT in this world, except for the small things in life: (a smile from a child, true friendship, real love, the beauty of nature, a flower, the stars at night, honesty, loyalty, generosity, humility, patience, truthfulness, gentleness, etc., etc.)

All those little things taste like the LIGHT, only that the LIGHT was like concentrating all those things in the same place at the same time. To tell you the truth, I could care less about money and stuff like that. Money is only something I need to survive physically (buy food, shelter, etc.). If I could eat air, I would not need money. (I am exaggerating a little, not much though!!! But I hope you get the idea).

Well, then I felt I was not allowed to "go" any further and I felt I was somehow "pushed back" very quickly (I guess it was like that), and very quickly I started to feel and see again my surroundings in the classroom. I could again feel the small annoyances of the physical world (gravity, the contact with my chair, etc.), my first reaction was to scream to my friends: "Hey, have you seen that light?!!!!!", well, let me say that better: actually, I believe the first thought I had was wondering whether they had also seen the light: "have they seen that light?" I just wondered if they had also seen it!

But when I turned to my right and left sides, everybody was doing just about the same thing as before (talking, playing, etc.). They showed no special reaction at all, so I understood (or assumed) they had not seen anything (but I never asked them), so I kept quiet (I was like when you are in love, just feeling and thinking about the nice, soft and WONDERFUL feeling of LOVE...and quietly enjoying it, like in a sacred atmosphere), the class continued, it ended. I went back to my house and I told nobody for many years. I didn't tell my parents, nor my brothers, nor my friends, nor my teachers, nobody!

During my whole life I have not been much interested in telling people about it. To me, it was simply an intimate experience that I had, and I know for sure that there are other WONDERFUL realities that we cannot see now with our physical eyes. I have not been very much interested in this issue for many years. I mean "interested" in the sense of telling others, because to me it was indeed the most important experience of my life. The LOVE the Light gave away makes you feel TOTALLY happy, and feeling you need nothing else AT ALL to be totally happy. Things of this material world cannot compare AT ALL to that type of happiness, (and I would write "AT ALL" with even bigger letters if I could).

Why was I not interested in telling others about it? For different reasons: I did not have any idea if anybody else in the world had experienced something similar, and I knew nobody in person. When I turned around 21 I learnt for the first time an experience similar to mine from the book "Life After Life" from Raymond Moody, (I read an article about him in the newspaper). That's the first time I became aware that something similar had happened before to other persons, but I had no idea how many. In fact, I thought very few people in the world had experienced it. When I turned around 17 years old, I started reading the Bible, and I was surprised to find out so many references about "the light of God", etc. Since then, I always interpreted those words ("the light of God") as something literal, as opposed to something symbolic.

In my case, the Light irradiated a feeling of PURE, PURE, PURE LOVE, which I considered to be a very intimate experience. Also, the first persons I told about it, my parents, (I told them when I was around 23 years old), did not have a good reaction. They looked at me funny, like saying: "Who knows what he saw!" I didn't like their reaction very much. I don't think they understood what I was talking about. Then I tried to tell a few other persons, but their reaction was also kind of neutral or even negative, and I quickly said to myself: "Forget it!, they'll never understand it and I won't be able to explain it to them." So, I decided it was not worthwhile sharing it, because it is totally impossible to transmit feelings or to put them into words.

But last year (starting February 2003). I have changed my mind. Why? Because I have found Internet web sites: and I have realized that there are many more persons than I had ever expected who have had similar experiences. I also read an article in The Lancet, I met other persons by e-mail (mainly from USA), and I learned a whole lot about this issue.

So, my position right now about this subject is the opposite than during all of my life. Now I have changed my mind and I do want to tell people about it. If they don't believe it, that's ok. If they think I am crazy, that's ok (I know I am not). I have realized that many other persons don't talk about this issue because they are kind of afraid about people's negative reactions, and that's why they keep it for themselves. I would also like to get in touch with other persons who have had similar experiences because, to tell you the truth, it is VERY frustrating talking to people who do not believe in these things.

(1963). (Cordoba). Spain.

When All Hope Was Gone

My life of forty-five years was
exceptionally busy. I had spent a better part
of a year trying to land a teaching position
since I had graduated from GVSU two
years before. Jobs were very difficult to find
in my area. I had to move again after only
three months. My cozy apartment building
had been sold and if I had been told it was
for sale, I would not have moved in.
Finances were a quite a challenge. I was
scarcely making it from week to week. Two
beautiful grandbabies were born eleven
days apart. One was unexpectedly born with
Down's syndrome. During the move I broke
my foot, so living in a new two-story
townhouse was somewhat of a struggle. As
the days passed, I wasn't feeling well. I felt
as though I was getting weaker and weaker.
I came down with laryngitis one day,
bronchitis the next, double pneumonia the
next, and six days later I was given a 5%
chance to live. My virus had gone into
sepsis, a poisoning of the blood. I acquired
toxic shock, which meant that all my organs
had shut down, along with a heart attack,
total life support and three weeks in a coma.
Later, on Mother's day, I had a stroke and
spent 43 days in the hospital. On April 24
my heart stopped, and I went to heaven. I

found out later it was the same day my father had died three years earlier.

God gave me a message and sent me home. He said, "You must tell the people. You must tell the people to stop going for the diamond and settle for the brass. Families who go for the diamond are workaholics, parents don't know their children and children don't know their parents. Families are breaking apart everywhere. You MUST tell them to stop going for the diamond." I then came back into my body. Heaven was a beautiful place. It was white, bright, sparkling, warm, safe, and good--all the positive adjectives one can think of. The greatest part of all was that I felt pure, sinless, flawlessâ€¦my slate was clean. My sins were completely forgiven.

After my visit to heaven I had a lot of spiritual warfare. One morning, at 3:00 a.m., I was too afraid to go to sleep. The spiritual warfare seemed to be continuous. I was so terrified I was afraid to close me eyes. I earnestly prayed for the Lord to send someone to pray with me. In a very short time, I saw a young man walk into my room. I wasn't sure if he was an angel or a real person. He asked me in a very kind voice, "How are you doing tonight?" I told him I was having a lot of spiritual warfare. He asked, "Can I pray with you?" I eagerly obliged and listened to a beautiful prayer. I felt the fear and tension leave my body starting at the top of my head and continuing to the bottom of my feet. I slept for four hours, which was the longest time I slept during my six-week stay at the hospital. The next morning as I was explaining to my friend what happened at 3:00 in the morning the same man walked into my room. I excitedly said to my friend, "Here comes my angel!" She replied, "He isn't an angel, he's your doctor!" I was pleasantly surprised that God had answered my prayer by sending someone to pray with me in addition to that, him being my doctor.

I have experienced many miracles during my healing. Since I was in a coma for 21 days, I was supposed to be in rehab for 21 weeks, but after a week of rehabilitation therapy they sent me home. Also, the doctors said that since I had kidney failure for so long I would either be on dialysis for the rest of my life or need a kidney transplant. My girlfriend, Bonnie, had already been checked to be a match for me. She was eager to give me one of her kidneys. My kidneys are now working well and there is no need for either one. Another miracle. My heart was also quite damaged, only working at 30% capacity, but before I left the hospital, it was working at 98%. I was given another blessing. My children were told I would be blind from the stroke. I had double vision for 3 months but now see better than I did before I was sick. Another miracle.

The night I was given a 3% chance to live, my friends and family were called in and the plans for my funeral were made. My girlfriend, Francine, wrote my eulogy. My friends, family, and pastor prayed over me. They were told all hope for me was gone. Even though the hope was gone, they still had not give up on me. They prayed over me through the night. In the morning I miraculously responded, to the amazement of the medical staff.

In January of this year, my sister, Brynn, called me from Florida. She told me she had a strong feeling something bad was going to happen. She thought our mom was going to become very ill. She bought a plane ticket for June 6th to come to Michigan. After I spent three weeks in a coma, I was then moved to general care. The following days my condition continued to improve dramatically. Two weeks after coming out of the coma, I spent a week in rehab and was then sent home to stay with my daughter. After a week, I was anxiously ready to go home after being away for six weeks. My first day home was June 6, the same day my sister arrived at the airport to come and help me for the next two weeks. I was strong enough to walk up to greet her at the airport. It was quite an emotional encounter. She was pleasantly surprised.

I have recovered 97%. I am getting singing andvoice therapy for the damage to my vocal cords due to being on the vent for three weeks. I also lost my hair four months after the incident, but it is growing back beautifully with many more curls than I have ever had before. I was blessed by obtaining a parapro position at the high school a mile from my home and love it. I am gaining more strength and endurance everyday. I now have a different outlook on life. In the past, I thrived on stress. I lived a life full of stress and often longed for more. Today, since I have been given a second chance on life and have been chosen by God to be His miracle, I am a different person. I enjoy sitting, talking, watching the beauty all around me. I have also taken up jogging 2 miles a day and love the energy it gives me. I have "de-stressed" my life in many ways. I now enjoy a life full of wonder, not of stress.

I am thankful for the experience of being so close to death. It has shown me the awesome power of prayer, and I was given the privilege to witness the answers to so many of them. It also showed me the

multitude of friends and family that were
able to stand in the gap to pray for me when
I could not, and I believe it is because of
them I am still on this earth. I have
immense gratitude to all of them. I have
also grown so much closer to my Lord. He
is with me each minute of the day. Through
Him, I experience life with such a grateful
attitude, almost as though I am experiencing
it for the first time.

Sandi

Nearly Drowned

This happened to me when I was a little boy, about 11 years old. We lived in a small town called Bennett, Texas and my father was on his vacation from work at the local brick manufacturing plant. One day during his vacation, he decided to go to the Brazos river to go fishing. The Brazos river was about five to seven miles from our house, so he drove to the river in our car.

Our next-door neighbor had three sons, one my age, one two years older, and one a year younger. Another neighbor two houses over had a single son who was two years younger than me. Since we all played together, I asked if they could all go with me and Dad to the river to go swimming.

All the parents agreed and we all piled into the car and rode to the river. Dad cast out his fishing gear and all of us boys put on our swimming trunks and went swimming a little way upstream from Dad, so as to not scare all the fish away from where Dad was fishing. After about a half hour of not catching any fish, Dad decided to move upstream to a different location. He told us to come upstream with him, so we told him we would wade upstream. He said OK, so

we started wading upstream while he
walked along the bank.

As we waded upstream, the others got about
40 feet ahead of me as I followed along.
Suddenly I went underwater! Over my
head! It happened so fast that I didn't have
time to catch my breath before going under.
I swallowed too much water. I surfaced and
began spitting water from my mouth, but
before I could gasp a breath of air, I went
under again and swallowed more water.
Again, I surfaced and began spitting water
from my mouth, but before I could gasp a
breath of air, I went under again and
swallowed more water. Now I am getting
desperate for air in my lungs! I thought to
myself, "I'm going to get a breath this time,
no matter what!" Again, I surfaced and
began spitting water from my mouth, but
before I could gasp a breath of air, I went
under again and swallowed more water.

Now, My stomach is hurting badly from
swallowing too much water. I told myself,
"I've got to stop swallowing all this water!"
But as I went under again, I swallowed
more water. Since I can't make myself take
a breath, and can't make myself stop
swallowing water, I'm getting extremely
exasperated and angry at myself! I am now
fighting as hard as possible to get above the
surface so I can get some desperate air! My

arm and leg muscles are getting dog tired from all of the struggling! I continued struggling my arms and legs, but now I became too exhausted. I thought to myself, "I'm too tired, I can't do any more. I quit."

Immediately, as soon as I quit struggling, everything seemed to go into slow motion. Just like you see in the movies and on TV, my struggles to get to the surface were in VERY slow motion. After what seemed an eon of struggling in slow motion, I started drifting upward. I continued to rise until I was about 12 or 15 feet above the water. I am really surprised! I'm up here and my body is still down there in the water, struggling! But I'm up here, and I don't hurt any more. I'm not gasping for air, nor hurting from all the swallowed water anymore. Everything is calm and peaceful up here. I'm OK!

After a little while, as I contemplated my situation, a sphere of light appeared before me about 20 feet in front of me. It was about the size of a basketball and gave off a very brilliant light. The sphere seemed to look like it had light inside that was churning. Churning like a thick cloud or smoke moving around, confined within the limits of the sphere. But it was light, not a cloud or smoke! For some reason, it seemed very important that I focus my attention on

it. As I watched it, a very black small dot
appeared in the center of the churning
sphere. As I looked at the dot, it suddenly
zoomed out and up toward me and there
stood the live figure of Jesus Christ in all
His splendorous glory!

Upon recognizing Him, I immediately flung
my arm up before my eyes and face and
told Him, "Get away! Get away! I'm not
worthy of being here with you!" He held
out His arm toward me and instantly, all my
fear went away. I looked at him and felt the
most overpowering sense of His love for
me. He stood before me and glorious light
emanated from Him in every direction. He
looked just like the pictures we see of him,
with the long hair and beard, and the white
wrapped cloth that was worn in His time on
earth 2000 years ago. Although His clothes
were white and his hair and beard was
black, he radiated light that was intensely
bright, and golden in color, and His
complexion appeared almost golden too.
The light was very, very bright, but it didn't
hurt my eyes. In the physical realm, it
would have blinded me, but here it was
normal.

The light emanated in every direction from
him, and I could see the rays as they flowed
from Him. Light travels at 196,000 feet per
second, but this light from him, I could see

it radiate toward me. I could see it leave
Him and move toward me. I could see it as
it went in every direction, and I know it
went FROM Him and outward until it
diminished. It seemed like my eyes were
now able to see things much more clearly.
Almost as if I was able to see
supernaturally, better than I had ever been
able to see before in the physical world. It's
like my vision could keep up with the speed
of light without any effort. As I felt the light
on me, I looked down at my body, and I
was also dressed in white, just like Him.
The wrapped cloth covered all of my body,
including my feet. Only my head was not
covered. With the light shining on me, I felt
the most overpowering feeling of love
flowing from Him to me.

He started talking to me, and I could hear
Him very clearly. I have always been hard
of hearing since infancy because of cerebral
palsy, the result of severe malnutrition. But
when He spoke, His voice was loud and
clear. His voice was so clear that it truly
sounded like music in my ears. Every
syllable rang with clarity, like a bell peeling
and reverberating through the air. Every
word sounded like a cascade of orchestrated
music. Now my hearing seemed to be
supernaturally better than I had ever been
able to hear in all my life. A strange thing,
though. When He spoke, His lips didn't

move. When I spoke, my lips didn't move. It's like we spoke to each other through extra-sensory perception. It seemed now like all my senses were supernaturally super sharp. It also seemed like I had suddenly gained supernatural wisdom. As He talked to me, I understood everything He said immediately. With my newly gained wisdom, I understood everything he said, no matter how complicated or complex. One thing that struck me was that when I spoke, He had already read my mind and knew what I was going to say. When He spoke, I had already read His mind too. I couldn't tell a lie, because as soon as I thought about what to tell Him, He already knew what I was thinking.

After conversing for a short while, a giant panoramic screen appeared. On the screen, different phases of my life history was being acted out in full 3-D living color. The actions being played out on the screen weren't in any chronological order, but every action or thought I had ever performed, or thought, during my short lifetime was there. You know the saying, "When a person dies, his whole life flashes before his eyes." Well, this is what was happening. Without pointing to any of the scenes, He asked me about one of the scenes. That scene in question immediately zoomed out big enough to cover most of the screen. I could see some of the other scenes still playing around the edges of our big scene, but they were in the background. He would ask me about something in this big scene we were viewing, and I had to explain to Him why I did or said the things that I had done or said in that historic moment of my life.

In one case, my twin sister and I were in a scene, and He asked me why I was pulling my sister's hair. In another case, why I lied to my mother. In another, why I was throwing rocks at my dog. In still another, why I wanted to fight and hurt my neighbor friend. In still another, why I was too lazy to do my homework that day. In each case, I first knew I had done something bad so I wanted to try to shade my answer a little so the effect wouldn't be so badly stated. As soon as I said it, He knew I wasn't telling the absolute truth and He severely rebuked me. After just two or three responses like that, and being severely rebuked, I knew I couldn't ever fool him, and for my own good I needed to come clean and tell the absolute truth.

In some scenes that were favorable to me, or in which I had done something good or outstanding, He praised me profoundly. In scenes that were funny, He laughed wholeheartedly with me. Did you know that

Jesus has the greatest sense of humor? After we had viewed and discussed most of the greatest or most important scenes, the screen went away.

After a short time it was time to go. He took my hand and we started traveling at a tremendous speed through a tunnel. Our feet weren't moving, nor were we in any kind of vehicle to carry us fast. We just levitated in mid air, and zoomed at a tremendous speed through the tunnel. As we moved through the tunnel, I knew we were going very, very fast. Strangely though, the walls, ceiling, and floor did not zoom past me in a blur like the case when speeding down the highway in a car. You know, how the scenery immediately by the highway will zoom past as we go down the road, but the scenery farther away from the highway moves by at a slower speed, so we can enjoy watching it go by. In this tunnel I could look at the wall, ceiling, or floor and it seemed to be moving right along with us at the same speed. The walls, ceiling, and floor of the tunnel seemed to be churning like smoke.

As far as I could see, ahead and behind, the surfaces were constantly churning. I like to think of it as firmament, for lack of a better word. Realizing that we had been moving for quite some time in this tunnel, I thought

"I wonder how much longer this will last?"
Looking ahead, I saw a light a long way
ahead. I knew that this was our destination
and was eagerly watching as we got closer
to the light.

Suddenly something physically hit my foot
as my body continued to struggle in the
water below, and immediately, I was back
inside my physical body. All the pain in my
muscles, stomach, lungs and throat was
thunderously evident and I was desperately
fighting to get to the surface again. James,
my neighbor swam underneath me and
came up between my legs and raised me up
until I surfaced and began gasping for air.
He then started swimming underwater with
me riding on his back. As he swam a little
way, I realized he was starting to struggle,
and I knew he needed air too.

Not wanting to drown him, I slid off his
back and stood up. I was now standing in
water chest deep, and James burst up
gasping for air. We waded to the bank and I
was too exhausted and collapsed. I
immediately vomited water. I vomited
again, and again, and again. But there was
no more water in my stomach. Yet I
continued to heave, again and again. Now I
was starting to get cramps in my stomach
from the dry heaving. Finally the heaving
tapered off and I was able to settle down

and rest. Immediately, Carl, the youngest
boy in our group yelled for help. He too,
now was drowning in the river. L. C., the
oldest boy in the group dove for him and
saved him.

Dad decided that we all needed to get home
now. There was too much happening too
quickly for comfort so we all loaded into
the car and came home. My body was very
sore for days after that. All my muscles
were sore, and my stomach hurt a week
from all the stretching it received because
of the excess water I had swallowed.

Because of all the excitement and shock of
the moment, the only thing I remembered
was the fact that my whole life flashed
before my eyes. I vividly remembered
seeing my life flash by, but I didn't
remember that Jesus was there too.

It wasn't until some twenty or more years
later that I started getting flashbacks and
slowly, over a period of time, I pieced
together the whole thing again.

HiRider

Love's Courageous Child

Cool website. I agree, the lasting impression
from an NDE is profound.

When I was 11 years old, I got a sore throat
that didn't go away and because I come
from a family of 10, going to the doctor was
a luxury. The sore throat, left untreated, was
discovered to be strep and since it cannot go
away with antibiotics, the strep infection
settled in my kidneys and I then had a
kidney infection/diseased called Nephritis
(Bright's Disease). The second night in the
hospital, I started to cry when my Mom and
Dad were going home after visiting,
because instinctively, I knew I would never
see them again. Because I was a kid, I knew
they were keeping this from me; however,
the body and the mind KNOW. They left
wondering why I was acting so strange.
Eleven year olds don't cry like that when
Mommy and Daddy leave. Well, at 11 p.m.
that night, the hospital called to tell my
parents that it wasn't likely that I would
survive the night. Last rites were given and
they monitored me all night, every 15
minutes.

In between the blood pressure monitorings,
I remember being in the corner of the room,

near the ceiling and looking down at my body as the nurse took my blood pressure. I wondered, hmmmmmmmmmm, what the heck am I doing down there? I'm obviously up here! Seemed strange, but I didn't worry about it. All of a sudden, there was a suction and I was moving through a tunnel at very, very, very high speed. When I came to an abrupt halt, I noticed 8 lighted beings off to my right and a big, beautiful white light directly in front of me.

Wow, I thought, and started heading towards that white light. I remember feeling a lot of peace, not sick, and the light seemed to have a "personality" or "essence" to it. It wasn't just a big 'ol floodlight. Felt great and I loved it. Just as I was walking towards the light, the lighted beings (angels--no wings) called me over to the side and told me to wait for a more superior being to arrive. I waited. The being arrived and then showed me part of my past and some of my future.

In particular, my little brother, Tim. Well, Tim is very hyper and a bit of a brat, so my response to the angels when shown some "footage" of Tim acting up and not being nice to me was, "Well, yea, Timmy's a brat." as if everyone in the Universe already knew that and there was nothing more to know. I was told by the angels, "Do not

make their problem, your problem, Dear
One." OK, I thought and thoughts are how
you communicate here, not voice. It didn't
make much sense, but OK. I was then asked
if I wanted to go into the light or back to the
body. This seemed like Sophie's Choice to
me, so I looked back down the tunnel and
then turned my head and back to the light,
back down the tunnel, back to the light,
back and forth, back and forth.

I understood that there were boundaries
there and that if I went into the light, I could
not come back and visa versa. I also
understood that what I could have there I
couldn't have here and what I could have
with my body, I couldn't have there. I was
told that I would be ill and that was not
negotiable. I was also told that they would
never leave me and all I had to do was ask
for their help and help would arrive. At that
point I said, "I want to live." and as I
finished the thought, I felt that same strong
suction grab me again and carry me back
down the tunnel. I did not re-enter the body
gently. It was like a big BAM! and I opened
my eyes and the nurse was standing next to
me taking my blood pressure ... again or
still? Well, I looked up at her and said, "I'm
going to be OK, now." She looked at me as
if I was delusional, but then I started
healing in leaps and bounds leaving the
docs and staff with their heads spinning.

I remember they wheeled me downstairs to get an EKG the next day and I thought, "You're a day late and a dollar short. It has been decided. I'm fine now." Well, the doctor didn't really understand why I was healing all of a sudden, but attributed it to the penicillin shot I got. I'm sure it helped, but well, no. He kept me there for 2 weeks and then released me. I healed completely, but at 31 years old, almost exactly 20 years later, I was diagnosed with a form of Muscular Dystrophy, which is incurable.

I remembered that I came back because in the moment I decided, I thought even if my body doesn't work quite right, I will always have the help of these angels and I want to come back for my shot at love. I understood that everything was worth it for love. I wanted it that much. Even though love was in the tunnel, clearly and abundantly, love with a body and in the physical world was a gift and I knew it and was willing to do so with a body that wouldn't work right. This was not negotiable. It was dictated to me and I needed to choose if I would return, not what kind of body I could return to.

Ironically, even though I was cured of the kidney disease one year later, the diagnosis 20 years later meant my family would be tested in ways I couldn't imagine. I always asked for help from my angels and I did not hide the fact that I believed in angels. This labeled me as "nuts" for my family to ridicule and my brother Tim and sister Jenny has refused to allow me to see their children. They don't want them to have "my influence." On Christmas, when I was in the hospital for surgery, they all brought me a figurine of an angel to the hospital, but then refused to let me see their kids.

Strange. So, the advice that the angels gave me, "Do not make their problem, your problem, Dear One." now makes sense to me, many, many, many years later. There have been days I have regretted choosing to come back, but overall, I am challenged to discover my place in this world and yes, I have been asked to marry. I have said no to all. They would have provided security, etc., but not the love I stood in when I went to that white light. I know that it is out there and I am not afraid of my family members telling me that I am some loser for not marrying.

When I go back to that tunnel with a white light, I do not want to have to say, "Yes, I know you taught me what love is when I was here last, but I had a little peer pressure, so I married Mr. OK. I didn't want to be the last kid to get married, you know." I can handle the ridicule. I want what I experienced in that tunnel with a white light

237

or nothing at all. I was a kid though, and acceptance of my illness and my body in this culture has been brutal. I have been told many reasons why I am ill ranging from "got myself sick (and supported by the Bible)." to I must have eaten the wrong foods, been depressed, or am trying to get attention.

None of the above are true and I don't feel the need to prove that to anyone. My values are different from my family's and when people meet me and my family, they swear I was not raised in the family I have. Some other guidance has been there.... healing me and loving me.

Love and Light, mnspiritsoars.

Election in Paradise

It was early April, 1981 during the preparation of Passover. An attempt had been made on President Regan's life a few days before. I was living on Stock Island in the Florida Keys at the time. At about eleven at night, I was compelled to fall on my face alone in the dark to pray on the floor. For three and one half hours, words rolled out of my mouth about every unkind thing I had ever done and every sin. I kept nothing secret and opened every darkest closet. Then for the next three and one half hours, words rolled off of my tongue about every dark and terrible act being committed among the nations of the earth. The floor was puddled with my tears.

With seemingly no strength left, I dragged myself onto the fold away bed in the living room and fell face up on it motionless. Just then, a beautiful place opened though the ceiling just like an ancient scroll opening with a living image of a beautiful green environment in it instead of script and I stepped though it into this place. I ascended a steep ridge effortlessly and all my senses were acutely functioning better than ever before. There were young hardwoods on the way up the ridge but at the top was a magnificent, spruce/fir/pine forest which seemed to have been given the utmost care. In front of me was a gorge and on the opposite side a great and wide waterfall which made yet a gentle wisp of sound because of the straightness of the gorge.

I stood frozen in awe. There were places to explore throughout the opposite side and everything was extremely well cared for. If this were not enough, a man in a long white robe emerged from a thick stand of firs farther down on the other side and walked across the gorge in the air without ever breaking stride or looking down. There was no bridge or fallen tree beneath his feet though I strained to see one. This man's gate was a noble gate and I immediately knew who it was without ever having been indoctrinated by religious orders or sects.

Still frozen in my tracks, he approached on a path which ran parallel to the edge of the gorge on my side cutting its way straight though the moss and young firs.

These words came from the depth of my spirit and I could not prevent them: I said, "Good morning, Precious-Wonderful Lord Jesus!" with the excitement of a little child who was receiving a thousand wonderful gifts at once. At this, The Light of The Eternal Father radiated from his heart and I

was enveloped and filled in the Light of
God. I asked him, "Is this the Light of the
Father?" and he replied, "It is as you say."
Then his eyes moved toward the gorge. I
followed them with mine and could see,
appearing out of the mist of the air, a golden
palatial structure. I asked, "Is this the
Father's House?" And he replied, "This is
the place we have prepared for you." Then I
asked, "Can I go over with you so that I
might meet the others who will be there?"
And He said, "No, it is not yet time. First,
you have much left to do." Then I said, "Let
me fly to the summit (on my side of the
gorge) and circle it three times and return
before you. Then let us embrace at length
before I must go." And he nodded saying,
"Go." I lifted into the air, the tips of the
spruces and firs passed beneath me at a
rough distance of fifteen feet, I circled the
summit and was then set back before him.
After a long embrace, I descended the ridge
eagerly toward my mission with full
knowledge I would return and that time was
no longer a concern.

At a halfway point along the descent, there
was a futuristic circular structure nestled in
a level area with every kind of hard and
softwood. The structure was filled with all
kinds of media, music and motion picture
equipment. Descending the ridge further, I
then returned to my body on the fold-up bed

which was miraculously kept alive with slow and shallow sinus rhythm and breathing.

I sprang up with a jolt glowing and bathing the room in white light. I was completely cleansed and as light as air in feeling. A golden sun had risen and my first act was to befriend a little child who was on his bike riding in circles alone beyond my front door. I put my hand on his shoulder, smiled and offered to show him how to play Yahtzee. Then I said: "If you believe you can roll five sixes, you will." On his first roll, five sixes stretched across the table close together in a straight line with all the dots pointing in the same direction. The next small miracle was when I wrote a spiritual song, "Glory To You, Lord", where a butterfly landed on the tuning keys of the guitar I was composing with. In the years to come, there were of course events, miracles and acts of far greater significance but this was the beginning as it happened.

For a long time, people from various places and walks reported that brilliant white light was radiating from me. Seven years before this 1981 event, my voice thundered saying that I stand on the stone of destiny and behold the wisdom of the ages. I knew it to involve the universe as well as the nations. Seven years after 1981 came the

Conservation Exchange* vision while I was managing at Bigelow Preserve. And seven years after that came confirmational visions that I had been given authority to address nations and worlds. There were also confirmations from spiritual leaders and spiritual people though the 1980s and 1990s who have been kept untarnished from the politics and meanderings of modern religions. I, myself, was kept safe by miraculous angelic intervention—and not only from this but from physical harms and discomforts along my journeys across North America. And some who were mean came to utter ruin overnight.

*Conservation Exchange is in fulfillment of the Prophet Isaiah. Global military forces and civilians work together in a Forest Recovery/Enhancement and Crops to End World Hunger Pact. Lasting global peace is achieved within a single year by common mission and no longer merely observed philosophically. That is just the beginning. Trillions in monetary units and resources otherwise earmarked for weapons and weapons platforms can then be ruddered to Advanced Individualized Education, Fuel-less Technology, Medical Cures, Affordable Energy and Environment Savvy Homes, Long Life Products/Materials, Major Costs and Tax Relief, The Needy and all people, environment and technological reformation programs that are designed to benefit all people/all life and to succeed. Rich or poor, we can no longer tolerate the violation to life, the natural wonders and the common liberty, happiness and well being of all.

How does this impact other worlds? It will become the universally accepted principle of right governance and the means though which peaceful open contact will occur. It takes all kinds of individuals to make this happen. The reward is that we will have overcome technological deprivation, wars, planetary devastation, disease, poverty and death itself under the most grueling of circumstances historically and will become a light indeed on the very Throne and Footstool of God: Earth. Once we were the children of God and now we become the light of God.

J. F.

(Seldom do I read such powerful script. This is more than a NDE, it is a transcendent NDE. Awesome, the last statement: "Once we were the children of God and now we become the light of God." Truly a nudge to get up and get going to make this a better world.)

Spiritual Encounter

The most important event of my life occurred in the early autumn of 1947 two weeks before my fourteenth birthday. If I had not experienced it and someone else told me this story, I would probably not believe it, so if any reader is skeptical, I will understand.

I was picking cotton on a plantation in northeastern Arkansas to earn money for school clothes. A neighbor of ours was transporting people from our area to and from the cottonfields about twenty miles from my home. There were about fifteen of us, I believe, from my age to elderly, working in the field that day. Among them my pal, Polly, a year older than I, and her mother and step-father.

Polly and I were picking a row each and a "snatch row" between us. That is, the two of us picked three rows as we went along. The one having her row ahead would pick the snatch row to keep all three rows even. Polly's parents were picking two rows each, as most of the workers were, so we soon pulled ahead of the others, giving us privacy for our conversation which we needed for it mostly concerned our plans for rebellion and living the life of a libertine.

After a bit Polly's parents scolded us for doing more talking than picking. Polly sassed back using profanity. Emboldened by her performance, I sassed too, but without profanity, as I had not picked up that habit. It wasn't done in our home. We did, however go to work in earnest because we knew we needed the money. We had about decided to use it for bus tickets to Texas to stay with a depraved uncle of Polly's who allegedly could get her a job singing on the radio.

We worked hard for awhile, Polly "walking" on her knees to save bending her back, and I standing bent over the rows, as I never was any good at picking from a kneeling position. When my back began to complain in earnest, I stood to give it a rest. It was a pleasantly warm, but not hot day with a clear blue sky dotted with a few small fair weather clouds. I think I was facing roughly northwest staring aimlessly into the blue and thinking of nothing that I recall, enjoying a gentle, refreshing breeze that began to blow over me ---- then THROUGH me!! Through every cell of me!! Cleansing me entirely. I have never in my life felt so clean, so refreshed.

And then HE spoke to me. I didn't hear a
voice nor see a form. But I was clearly and
intensely aware of a communication
directly into my consciousness from an
OTHER of indescribable goodness,
kindness and power, and I recognized Him
as I would my mother or father. I felt I had
known him before but had somehow
forgotten him until that minute. I trusted
him completely with no apprehension for he
was, I knew, completely to be trusted.

Here, as nearly as I can express it in the
clumsy medium of language, is the content
of that communication:

I was made aware that sin was destroying
me. I was shown the image of a form, that
as I recall it seems now to have somewhat
resembled a fetus (though at the time I had
no idea what a fetus looked like) which I
understood was myself. It was being eaten
away by a horrible sore, disgusting and
revolting in the extreme. I was made to
know that He felt great sorrow for this state
of affairs. He told me that if I would choose
a path characterized by love and peace that
he would be with me to guide me all the
way and at the end of the path I would come
to him. I was shown an image of a path
through a wood and a light like a spotlight
shining down upon it ahead of me. Then
when he spoke of my coming to him I was

caught up into the midst of a glorious
golden light; suspended there, embraced in
perfect love and peace and joy beyond
expression, the joy of coming home at last.
For this destiny I had been created.

Suddenly I was back in the cotton patch just
as before, except my face was wet with
tears. I was so terribly sorry for every
unkind thing I had ever said or done. I felt a
deep love for all people and a feeling of
how infinitely precious each person is. I
looked at Polly kneeling between the cotton
rows looking up at me and her face was wet
with tears as well. We had apparently had
the same or very similar experience.

The first thing we did was to run back to
where her parents were working and try to
tell them what had happened and to
apologize from our hearts for the way we
had so recently spoken to them. The next
Sunday we astonished everyone by
appearing in church.

I have, over the ensuing years, considered
many "explanations" for this event, and can
honestly find none more believable than the
one I unquestionably accepted at the time;
We had an encounter with the living God.

M. B.

An Entity of Love

I was seventeen years old in 1989 and had
mistakenly mixed the wrong medications
together which I found out later can cause
heart arrhythmia or affect the heart. I had
been having serious problems with acute
bronchitis and already was having major
difficulties breathing anyway. I had been
bedridden for a few days and my friend
Jane was with me when this happened,
because she lived with me and my mom at
the time.

She had been reading to me to cheer me up
next to my bed. All of a sudden it was like I
had this profound calmness or sense that I
was about to die, to this day I don't know
how I knew that. Suddenly right after that I
remember feeling my chest flooded with
what I can only describe as tightness, like
an intense tightness as if something was
squeezing me on the inside, but it didn't
actually hurt, it just felt very strange.

Then it felt like I was tilting somehow (even
though I was just lying down) and I recall
feeling as if I was falling into some
darkness. The next part, if anyone can
understand this, I remember with a different
kind of memory, like it was imprinted on
my deepest sense of self. There was only
what I can describe as a churning blackness,

like black walls that were soft but very
thick, moving, but gently.

Then there was this little bright circle that
kept getting bigger and larger and then it
was like I was floating into this really
bright, and I mean incredibly white lighted
atmosphere where I could not see anything,
even though I could still "see".

The only scary part of this whole
experience was when this bizarre "thing"
appeared and started reaching for me and
seemed to howl like it was going to devour
me and then bam! It was like something
incredibly powerful scooped me up and
whisked me away from this evil thing and
that's when I experienced what I think was
God or Jesus or some kind of awesome
entity.

The weird part is, I distinctly felt that this
entity changed from an array of lights and
moving texture to a form of a more
recognizable person. But it was not a
person. That's what was so weird. It was
like I could tell that the 'entity' was
attempting to comfort me by appearing in a
form I felt comfortable with. Then I
remember feeling that we could talk without
words, like we were communicating
instantly and 'it' understood literally every
single nuance of my character, my feelings,

my entire being. I felt like I was in the presence of a parental type entity that was so incredibly WISE and so amazingly patient and loving and kind.

I felt the fastest flash of the events of my life and then the entity 'spoke' and said "You have to go back, it's not your time yet" even though I only 'sensed' the words. I distinctly remember begging not to go and then actually arguing with it, but not in an impolite or angry way, just insisting that I do not want to go back, and that I wanted to stay with 'it'. I swear, I felt like a little kid with this entity, but at the same time a little selfish because when I was with 'it', I felt so much peace and sanctuary and love and stability.

Anon

"Home, I'm Going Home"

Tuesday, May 17, 2005

In 1961 at age seventeen I went to bed a cheerful, atheist, school girl.

Hours later I was slowly waking up due to feelings of intense joy, speeding forward, sitting up with my legs crossed. The faster I went the more intense the feelings became and I was totally awake in inky darkness absolutely overcome with complete joy.

Then I knew, "HOME, I'm going HOME." I was amazed, "How did I know that? If I had ever been here before I would have remembered this! I never would have forgotten about this." The faster I went the more excited I became. Then I realized I was finally awake. I had woken up. My whole life I had been asleep.

This was astonishing as I had always thought I was awake in life and now knew I was finally, gloriously awake. There is no memory of my arrival here. Almost as if my memory was blacked out. I was standing in a white robe looking downward while three men wearing glowing robes were discussing me. I think they had been talking to me. I was absolutely and completely, joyously content to be with them. Not anyone I knew and yet I am positive I did know them and they certainly knew me.

Number one said, "She doesn't need this anymore," and reached into the top of my head and pulled out a two or three inch wide, dirty grey gauzy strip of material. About five feet long. Exactly my height. He threw it away and number two said, "Well, she doesn't need this either," and pulled out another long, dirty strip. They all proceeded to take out maybe four to six more strips. I was being relieved of what I had picked up in life that was destructive and needed no more. Almost as if I were cleaned from the top of my head to the bottom of my feet. Untruths I had believed in absolutely were simply thrown away.

I do not know how I arrived here. I know I was no longer in a body form. I was instead an oval shape and yet still very much me. There were others just like me. All exactly alike. Maybe one hundred, maybe ten thousand. We were all sitting side by side in many, many rows. The same, all the same being made of the same universal stuff.

We were all part of and partaking of this. This is difficult for me to tell. I can't begin to put into words anything about this that would even be close to the reality. I was facing Jesus Christ, above me and directly in front of all, seated on a huge throne. The massive wave like pulsations were all around us and through us. We were covered with and in side of this, ineffable, ineffable, I don't know. This is what is. This is so overwhelming even now that I want to throw my self on the ground and sob for the loss of this. This is what is, all there is, we are of this and we are here now with and for this.

Then I had the thought, "I was in back, not the front, not close to him as the others were," and I became angry, furious even, as a little child being kept from what she needed and I said, "Why not me? They all get close, I never have what others have."

Before the thought was finished I was a foot away from Jesus, face to face, next to him with his eyes staring into me, yet still where I was with the others. He told me, "You have everything that everyone else has. All have the same." I was again enfolded in the pulsations.

A figure, a man touched me from behind on my right shoulder and said, "You have to go back now." I heard it and ignored it. He tapped me and repeated it. I yelled, "No!" I knew I would never go back. I was where I belonged and was staying. I had been there and it was over. Now I was home with Jesus and would never again go back.

Someone took my shoulders and began pulling me away and I began fighting harder and harder and screaming, "no", but they were completely calm and at peace as they threw me backwards and down. I slammed into my body, landing on my back and laid there horrified at what had happened.

I opened my eyes and saw the ceiling and the closet of my bedroom. I lay there filled with despair and horror. I had been thrown out. Thrown out, and the desolation was deep and terrible.

The alarm clock went off and I stood up and stared at my open palms, shaking, thinking, "I'm back, oooh, I'm back, I'm really here." I dressed, ate, got my books and went to school as if it never took place. But, Oh, it did. It was always with me, but never admitted, which was strange because it seems now, as if it was always right in my face while I denied it.

Looking back now I see I was in a state of shock for many years. I had been thrown back, tossed away, completely changed and nothing fit anymore. There were no answers

anywhere because it was 1961 and the
questions weren't even asked. It didn't
happen because it didn't exist.

The world I came back to was
incomprehensible. People lied and I
watched and was shocked. "Why is he lying
to her? They both know she can see through
him". But she didn't and I didn't know why.

I was lost and I left home because I could
not fit in anymore. What was important
before was less than nothing now. What
was important I could not speak of without
being considered psychotic. According to
my psychology classes I evidently was
schizophrenic, but it didn't seem so. And yet
I knew I had left my body and gone
somewhere else, even worse, I wanted to
leave this world again and go back. Yet I
was very calm, there didn't seem to be much
to be upset over.

I did have times of tremendous peace and
moments of knowing, at times almost as if
there was someone unseen at my side.
Oops, psychotic again.

I haunted book stores and libraries, thinking
someone must know what happened, what
this is, but I never even got close to an
answer. My life became a roller coaster.

In 1970 I found Emerson's Essay's. It was
clear he knew. I read his essay's over and
over again trying to feel home once more.
That was a start. Then Jane Roberts and
Seth surfaced. More information! At last I
was learning something. I found Richie's
book of his experience and recognized what
had happened to me. His book was a life
line.

I had not died and I had no life review, but
oh, the changes it had made in me. I came
back stripped of any ability to hide my
thoughts or attitudes. Indeed I found it
difficult to lie, believing people could see
through me. That all was known. I had a
tremendous thirst for information about
almost everything. There was still
something in my hands and I would look at
my palms and not know what to do with
them. But there was something there, there
still is, but what? What was I supposed to
do? I don't know. I knew things I shouldn't
and began to get what I call packages of
information if I was curious enough to open
them. And I was always curious.

I was called naive and thought to be a
dummy because I didn't understand what
was simple to others. Yet I excelled in
school and it became a lark. Strange events
took place around me, physical events
happened that don't happen. I began to see

dead people whom I knew and a few I didn't
know.

I found Robert Monroe, Moody, Betty Edie
and the rest, I began to mention it to my
husband. The poor man was very worried
about me. So I told my best friend and she
tried to believe me so I made her read the
books. Only five people know, so this is my
debut. I am hoping I will have fulfilled what
ever I am supposed to do. You` see, I still
don't know. The only ones who can know
are those who have experienced it.

They are the only ones I accept any
information from any more. I am done
listening to experts who never experienced
anything. Their theories may sound great,
even learned, but they aren't even in the ball
park because they don't know where it is.

Thanks and blessings to all of you who have
told your stories. They have been many,
many lifelines to me. Maybe I will be a help
to someone. Meet you in the great beyond
folks, because for certain that's where we
will all be.

J.S.

Jesus with the Biggest Smile

This is not my nde account, but that of a friend's told to me over 30 years ago, and still fresh in my memory.

My friend had been in a car accident that sent her face through the windshield, and back out again. She was on the operating table when she died for about 5 minutes. She said she felt herself leave her body and was looking down at all the chaos going on and wondered who was that bloody mess lying on the table. It took her a while to realize it was her body, as she was watching all of this from the celling at the time. She then floated to a waiting room where she saw her family gathered and obviously very upset at the situation at hand. Her mother and father were crying, and she kept telling them she was ok but wasn't getting a response.

Then she said she went through the ceiling of that room and through the floors of the hospital to being outside and speeding towards the night sky. She passed planets and stars with great speed and found herself surrounded by all kinds of beautiful colors that she said were not like colors here on earth. She didn't have time to be scared, being enthralled by all she was seeing in this spectrum of colors. She then found herself going towards a bright light and when she got close to it she said there was Jesus with the biggest smile on His face and it was the most beautiful face she had ever seen. She said His hair was auburn and His eyes were green and His complexion was olive colored and before she could stop herself she said "Oh my God it's Jesus Christ"! Now you would have to know this woman to understand this being funny because she was the type of person who said "Oh my God" all the time. She said there was so much love radiating from Him that she wanted to stay in His presence forever. He then asked her telepathically if she wanted to stay, and of course she said "yes" but can I just go back to tell my parents I'm ok because they are very upset right now. With that thought she was back in her body and woke up three days later while it was raining outside and she said she had never seen the trees look more beautiful with the rain dripping from them and was very thankful to be alive.

Needless to say so were her parents thankful, but when she tried to tell them about meeting Jesus, of course they said it was just a dream or hallucination from the drugs given to her in surgery. She then told them about visiting the waiting room and was correct with naming all the people that were anxiously waiting to hear if she was going to live or not. This her parents had no explanation for, so they just told her to forget about it.

When her pastor visited, she gave it one more shot in telling him about it, thinking if anyone will believe me he will. Well he didn't believe her and said she shouldn't be saying such things because it was all just a reaction to the drugs, and if she continued to insist she would probably have to see a shrink because she was not dealing with the trauma, and losing touch with reality.

So needless to say she kept her mouth shut, but knew beyond a shadow of a doubt that what happened to her was real. She only spoke of it to people like myself whom she knew had an open mind and would not say it was from severe head trauma and many meds.

It took her a year to mend with more reconstructive surgeries and her memory was poor during this time, but when it came to that ride, a word of it never changed and she recalled it with no trouble at all. I for one believe her without a shred of doubt. And if you heard her tell it you would be crying right now because it was just that powerful and beautiful and I knew it was the absolute truth.

Jesus is real, folks. - T.

I was Shot in the Head

I have not really talked about it much since it happened, but about five years ago I got shot in the head and died. I seen things that I can't explain, things I always sat at home and thought would never happen to me.

After being shot in the head, I was left for dead. I can still today count how many times I ever asked the Lord for anything, and that was one of those times. I asked not to be taken from my family, my wife and kids. I was able to drive about three miles for help and while I was laying beside my truck in a pool of blood I had someone to help me, I think an angel. When the ambulance arrived one of the medics said my head was being held up in a manner he didn't understand. As I watched them put me in the ambulance, I heard a voice that sounded like no man or woman and had a taste in my mouth that was sweeter than sweet.

Telling this story sounds so silly, but that's what I always thought about all of the shows I used to watch about others being shot. I just thought it would never happen to me.

One other thing I'm wondering about, it
might be wrong, I'm happy to be alive
today, but when I think back to that day I'm
more mad at the doctor who saved me than
the guy who shot me.

Doesn't make any sense does it. Please
write back if possible.

S.N.

*(It does make sense to a near death
experiencer, and he was emailed back.)*

We Missed the Bridge

After drinking half a bottle of Tequila, and
half a bottle of some cheap wine, by myself,
(I forget the proof now, but a high alcohol
content) and smoking a few joints of pot, on
an empty stomach, three young men and I (I
had a crush on one of them) got into another
guy's car (one of the three I was with) to
drive me home.

I was already very late for dinner. I had
turned 15-years-old the month before, and
had been hanging out at the local shopping
center with "friends." We were driving on
an old country road, speed limit was 45
mph, but we were going 75mph. Coming
around a curve at that speed, there was a
one-lane bridge we didn't know about. We
missed the bridge completely, flew off the
road and bounced off three trees. One on
each side, and came to a stop at one front
and center, down in a deep ditch.

The three boys walked away, supposedly
dazed, I guess they went home. (I was told a
few different stories at this point, I was
unconscious at the time). The driver of the
car, went home and told his mom that he
killed a girl (me) and to call the police.

That's only one version I've heard, maybe I'll never know, anyway, back to the story!

I was left in the car, on the back floor, they thought I was dead, for approximately 20 minutes, (that's what I heard), before any rescue personnel found me. I went in and out of consciousness in the ambulance. (There is another story behind that -- nightmares that lasted 6 months to a year after the accident). I "saw" the doctors and nurses trying to save my life, from above the operating table. My dad had instinctively followed the ambulance from the highway to the hospital (he wasn't sure if it was me, but, knew it).

They wouldn't let my parents see me, there wasn't time, then, they had to rush me in another ambulance to a different hospital because the first one didn't have the right equipment to keep me alive. That's the first time my parents saw it was me, only briefly. I was in Intensive Care for three weeks, fighting for my life, I suppose.

At what point I died, I'm not really sure. I went down a long dark tunnel, faster than the speed of light, though it seemed to take a long time. I saw a light at the end of the tunnel and when I got there, as I passed through the golden gates. (I'm shaking now as I write). There were people, relatives I had never met and others, beckoning me to come in, smiling, happy, loving. (I'm about to cry, but, I'll go on). Just as I was going through the gates, A HUGE hand came out of the blackness to swoop me up, I was as tiny in this gigantic palm as a dot, to bring me lovingly, gently, back to my hospital bed. I guess it was then that I awoke from my coma, with my parents by my bed.

The first question I asked, as best I could, was "What time is it?" My parents were overjoyed, and they told me it was July 31st -- six weeks I was unconscience! My dad asked if they could get me ANYTHING at all... I answered "ice-cream," my mouth was so dry! They couldn't understand me yet, so, they said to try to name something similar (or, something like that) and I thought, then said, "freezer." I was SO happy that they could understand that, and they put it all together and finally guessed what it was that I wanted!!

Then, I had three weeks of intensive therapy, occupational and physical, to learn how to read, write, walk, talk, everything, all over again. (I'm shivering now)! Okay, back to my story. I had to have two months of home-teaching my 10th grade year, as I couldn't get on a school bus with a full-length leg-cast. I broke my right leg, left thumb at the base, and one of my collar

bones. I had a mid-brain concussion, and
came close to being permanently brain-
damaged. My left arm had covered my heart
and stayed like that, until a therapist
gradually worked it down so that I could
use my arm and hand again.

Wow!! That didn't take TOO long, did it?
I'm breathing a sigh of relief, now...I'm
drained.

D.

A New Hope

Following my accident when I was severely burnt, my last memory was being injected morphine at Staincliffe Hospital, Dewsbury, the place I was born and nearly died; following this I was rushed to Pinderfields Hospital at Wakefield where I was to spend the most painful 13 weeks of my life.

My next memory was awakening and finding me stood in a darkened room and in the far corner was a bed, to which all sorts of electronic equipment were attached beeping away and in the bed seemed to be a person but I just wanted to get away from the place.

Strangely all the pain I had previously suffered was gone like one big nightmare, I remember in my disorientated state somehow leaving the room, into a long deserted corridor, illuminated sparsely with a few night lights.

As I approached the end of the corridor a nurse came out of a nearby staff room, laughing merrily at some joke her and the rest of the staff must have been sharing, as she turned and walked towards me I just froze, however, her eyes showed no

acknowledgment of my physical presence
as she passed by me.

I called out to her when she was about 15
feet past me but she showed no signs of
either seeing me or hearing me, I thought
this was a little weird by now, but my
instincts told me to find an outside door and
get away from this strange place.

After a while traveling through the maze of
corridors I found a locked exit, upon trying
the door to my amazement I found my hand
just passed right through it and to my utter
bewilderment I found I could walk right
through it, I could feel no warmth or cold, I
seemed to myself what I can only describe
as a physical point in space that could see
and hear but could not interact.

With further astonishment I now found
myself perhaps 150 foot up in the air and
heading through the night, below I could
see the tops of the street lamps and a few
cars wondering around, I distinctly
remember flying over a railway viaduct and
towards the city of Wakefield.

The neon sign over the nightclub called
Rooftop Gardens drew me like a magnet
being familiar with the place during my
many nights out with my friends, The

Gangster and The Savage One, I must of
thought in retrospect that a familiar place
would relieve me of all this craziness but I
was flying for Gods sake.

I came down to land near the entrance to the
club in front of two of the bouncers I
remembered from yesteryear. I had on
many occasions in the past greeted these
two individuals, however on this occasion
they just continued their small talk
oblivious to my sudden appearance from the
night sky.

I paused to think and reached out with my
hand to touch a nearby wall that was
adjacent to the clubs entrance but my hand
appeared to have no physical substance and
just passed into the fabric of the wall.

It was now that the awful truth finally
dawned on me. The people were unable to
see or hear me, The wall, The doors to the
hospital, just suppose they were perfectly
normal? Just suppose that it was me who
had changed? What if for example I had
somehow lost my "hardness", my ability to
grasp things, even, to make contact with the
world -- even to be seen?

I mean what is the point in going anywhere
if, as the final shreds of my rational mind
pointed out, if you cannot be seen, and what

was that mound in that bed in the little
hospital room I had left could that have
been my physical body?

I didn't like this line of thought, a human
being is not separated from his body unless
he is dead, then what state was I in now? It
can go through doors without opening them,
it can fly like a bird, it does not feel cold or
warmth, and remarkable these qualities are,
they are no good if one cannot be seen. I
decided at this point to go back to
Pinderfields and see if I could reacquaint
myself with my body, surely pain is better
than this.

No sooner had this thought occurred to me I
found myself moving at incredible speed
through the night back to the doors of
Pinderfields, it seems in this strange state
you travel by thought alone, handy this may
be, but the novelty soon wears off rapidly.

Now Pinderfields is a big hospital and in
my rush to get out of there I had forgotten
just where I had left my body (or indeed
what was left of it by now).

I just didn't have a clue which room it
was in. I rationalised that it must be
somewhere in the burns unit, but it was no

use asking the doctors or nurses because
they couldn't see me or hear me.

After an extensive search I managed to find
the burns unit, and by wandering from room
to room I finally found the room I had left
earlier, and there I was lying unconscious,
wired up to an whole variety of strange
gadgets.

At this point out of pure desperation for
something to do, I decided to recite the
lordâ€™s prayer something I had learnt
many years ago at school.

The very next moment the absolute
impossible happened; a tiny pinprick of
light at the side of the bed began to grow
brighter and brighter, at first not noticing
the pin prick of light I thought it was a tiny
night light that was the rooms only
illumination that was getting brighter.

But then I saw it was coming from beside
the white bedside table at the head of the
bed, it continued to brighten as I watched, it
brightened to such an extent that had it been
any ordinary light I would most certainly of
been blinded.

The next moment there flooded directly into
my mind the words "Stand Up...you are
now in the presence of the Son of God",

whereupon out of the light stepped what I could only describe as the most magnificent Being I have ever known.

Thankful at last for a little company in this strange situation I joked "That's it!...Just like that...I am with the Son of God...Isn't there a reception area or something before we meet?"

I felt a presence of Power and pure Love that was older than time but yet more modern than anyone I have ever met.

In the first stage of my experience, what I can only refer to as the earthbound state, I had lost three of my senses; smell, taste, and touch, however in this further stage in the light, time disappeared completely, a bit like in a dream, and I was aware of all my thoughts and actions in my life up to the present day as one big whole.

Every moment in my life was recurring before me at once, and the same instant as part of some enormous four dimensional sight and sound mural.

I guessed this was my life review.

But emanating from the Being projected pure love, up to that point in my life I had

come across much laid-back always
blaming anyone and everyone for the results
of my actions.

I also saw from a further dimension an
observation of my interactions with others
from the other persons point. I also saw
parts of the future which was hazy, however
I distinctly remember being told that a girl I
had met but would never marry had an
important role in the creation of my son
who was very special. I saw all of my
educational achievements so far were
purely superfluous, but it was the way I
treated others that was important, and I
could see the consequences of my lack of
interactions with my fellow students at
York University (which I had luckily just
graduated a month before).

I could see how the other students saw me
as weird and very anti-social, and they tried
to avoid me where possible so that they
could avoid the negative effect I had on
them, hence leading to a deeper feeling of
depression thus increasing my isolation.

An endless viscous circle that had
dominated my life.

I even could see the hurt on my best friend
-- The Gangsters emotions when he pulled a
bird called Cherelle at Rooftop Gardens,

but, I had done my best to split them up by
pouring a pint of lager on her head and
being very rude.

The tapestry of life was in front of me, and I
could see how my decisions now, would
effect the future. All of my ambitions of
being wealthy and having many material
possessions was regarded by the Being of
light with as much distaste as was my lack
of enthusiasm for interacting with my
fellow men.

I could see how my life would change, and
where I had once sought money and
possessions, I now treasured simply making
other peoples lives more pleasurable at the
expense of my own well being.

The Being of light then turned to me and
said via thought dynamics "Michael, What
have you done with your life so far?" I
replied using my mind: "Why didn't
someone tell me this was what life is
about?" The Being replied "Somebody did
nearly 2000 years ago in your linear time --
Me!"

I suddenly found myself on the move again,
this time we didn't bother about doors it was
straight up through the hospital roof, then
we flew at incredible speeds across the

surface of the earth, however there was no wind to slow us, and just a few moments later I found myself approaching a city beside a huge expanse of water.

In the city all the streets and offices were unbelievably crowded, and I could see people passing through other people like they wasn't there.

We walked into a factory and I saw assembly line workers who were putting together lawnmowers enjoying a coffee break while behind them a woman was pleading for a drag of their cigarette as through she wanted it more than anything in the world.

When one of the workers clearly blind and deaf to the women behind him actually took a cigarette out of his packet and began to smoke it, the woman repeatedly snatched at it, but it was as if she was clawing at thin air.

I came to the conclusion that those people must be ghosts, even though they were dead, they remained chained to the material world by the very things they had deemed most important during their lifetimes, their jobs, their cigarette smoking, their material possessions.

Myself and the Being of light moved from city to city visiting endless places he had to show to me, in one house, I remember a younger man followed an older man from room to room saying "I am sorry dad!," he kept saying repeatedly "I did not know it would do this to my mum -- I just didn't understand!"

The older man was carrying a tray filled with tea and toast into a room where a clearly unwell elderly lady was sat up in bed. "I AM SORRY" the younger man cried in frustration over and over again, but clearly his agony fell on deaf ears.

"Why is he so sorry?" I enquired to the Being of light, referring to the younger man's pleas. "He committed the ultimate selfish act" said the Being touching his long beard, "suicide." He continued with tears welling in the corner of his eyes "and chained to every consequence of their act of cowardice they are well and truly earthbound" he finished, but I knew the answer before I asked.

My next visit was back to the night club in Wakefield called Rooftop Gardens where I had visited earlier in my disorientated state, but without the concept of time, earlier and later were meaningless, it is a bit like telling someone blind from birth what it is like to see.

Inside the nightclub was an impossibly crowded place where I watched ghost alcoholics mingling with living drunks, and whenever a drunk lapsed into a drunken stupor a desperately thirsty ghost sprang inside his body so that the two became one.

The living could be distinguished from the ghosts by a faint cocoon of light around them, however when any living being became inebriated their light cocoon faded, enabling one of the many hovering ghosts to take over their body and literally possess the person.

So horrific was the scene that the only words in my mind that could describe this was "hell."

The mingling ghosts with their eyes so set on alcohol desperately clutching at real life beer glasses had blinded themselves to the magnificent Being that accompanied me -- Indeed the Being told me to keep my eyes firmly on him -- probably he was aware of my past record.

In this world of thought far beyond space and time (Thought is a more fundamental principle than the illusion of space or time

which pale into mere shadows) it can
seemingly be either heaven or hell of your
own making.

Earthbound ghosts destroyed by hatred,
lust, and destructive thought patterns, find
that whatever they think, however fleetingly
or unwittingly became instantly apparent to
all those who are around them, and more
completely than words could have
expressed it, and much faster than sound
waves could of carried it.

The thoughts most commonly
communicated amongst earthbound spirits
was usually selfish thoughts and this by its
very act kept the being earthbound, the
Being of light it seemed felt only
compassion for these unfortunate souls but
he knew it was their will not his that kept
them there.

I felt like Scrooge in "The Christmas Carol"
having this wise Being accompany me back
to the hospital for the final time, I wanted to
start my life again afresh when I would care
far more about other people and not just
myself.

No longer would money and possessions be
my supreme objective, but I would live my
life with a desire to make other people

happy -- the old "Mad Mick" was truly
dead, and the new one ready for a
reincarnation.

We entered the hospital room for the final
time, and the image of the being and the bed
before me faded -- the walls that surrounded
my little room at Pinderfields became solid
again, it was early morning, and I was
informed by a nurse who had come in to
open the curtains that it was two days since
my accident.

The pain was still there, but somewhat
dulled by the drugs I had been given. It was
to be another thirteen weeks before I was
released and I had many more strange
experiences in there, but nothing that could
be compared to the one I have shared with
you all.

After subsequent research into my favourite
subject -- Physics -- I have found that with
the merging of two theories of the universe,
Quantum Mechanics and General
Relativity, it appears that the three
dimensions of space and one dimension of
time is in fact an illusion created by the
world of thought.

Spirits who remain earthbound do
eventually find that hatred and envy are the
very emotions that keep them there, but

wouldn't it be easier to help our fellow
human beings while we are alive.

"Lay not up for yourselves treasures on
earth" -- Jesus

Michael.
A New Hope

The Day That Lives Forever!

"A Journey From Faith To Knowing!"

The Life After Death experience of L. F. in the year of Our Lord 1963.

It was 1963. I was to be discharged from the Navy in October. After two tours "In Country" it was great getting back to "The World." I had cash in my pockets, friends on the Beach, places to go and women to meet. California, what a place to wait out the time to discharge. I wanted a car to drive across the states on my way back home and being a Ford owner all of my short life, I decided to get the brand new, never before shown model of the up and coming 64 Mustang.

They normally come out in the Sept-Oct. months, but for some unforeseen reason, this year they came out early and were sold as 63.5 models because it came out in May. I saw it, I loved it, I bought it! It was a 289HPCI Fastback, Competition Yellow 5spd. Wood trim interior, leather seats with galloping mustangs across the bucket seats and a full floor console. What a beauty and Really Fassssst. We [the "Stang" and I] were the hit of N.A.S. LeMoore.

There was a huge "going away party" for a friend of mine, off base, and I was running late. Several of the girls called the base to see what was keeping me and I told them I'd be headed out shortly. I jumped in the "Stang" and bolted out the gates headed to town on a clear, warm California night. The road was a two lane Highway almost "straight arrow" most of the way into town and I started to pour it on to make up time. There was no one on the road, no lights coming or going and I was doing 100+mph, just humming along. Had the Radio blasting, looking in my rear view mirror at the "Cutsie" stuffed Tiger resting in the back window, no cops, no worries and nothing but a good night on my mind. The road was flying by, the white dashes were almost a solid line and the world was mine. I was young, popular, educated and soon to be discharged like my friend tonight. What a great feeling.

I looked at the road ahead and for no reason at all I saw the front end of my car nose down and there were thousands of sparks flying past the fenders, they were beautiful sparkles of light flowing past the windshield with particules of blue, reds, and greens. It was a magnificent sight against the darkening skyline. At first I thought I had blown the engine, but all the smoke and flames seemed to be coming up from the sides, where the wheels should have been and the increasing torrent of shimmering streams of rhinestone, crossing both fenders, appeared as a welder frantically sharpening the edge of a fine sword. Through all the smoke and sparks bellowing in front of me, some coming through the windows, I looked further down the road I was now tearing up at a frantic pace, and saw, in the far distance, a set of headlights coming in my direction. Just a pin prick of light mind you, but getting brighter and stronger as I careened toward them and them toward me. I thought to myself, "Wow, are these people gonna really see something strange when I finally come to a stop. I must look like a Roman Candle right about now to them."

Just then the front end dug into the asphalt like a sharpened spade through hard, dried and crusted earth in the desert landscape, and in what was less then a second, the "Stang" flipped head-over-heels, becoming completely airborne, and I felt myself coming out of the seat and hanging in mid-air, as the entire car rotated around me. In what I thought took minutes, I found myself upside down in the interior of the car, with my head where my feet used to be and my right shoulder was pinned against the center console, my head imprinting the chrome stick shift. I thought to myself: WOW, this

is gonna hurt when we [the Stang & I]
finally touch down, but for now both of us
were as weightless as astronauts rocketing
through the blackness of deep space: Then
we did [land] and it did [hurt] but now the
car went from the head-over-heel flip, to
long and furious barrel rolls, end over end,
again and again, and with every one I would
crash my head and shoulder into the center
console and shiftier. I could feel the broken
glass from all the windows exploding with
every landing. So as not to slip into
unconsciousness, I managed to count
everyone of those flips, thinking the last one
I counted would be the Last One I'd have to
count, but it took NINE of those babies to
finally lose all the momentum necessary to
bring us to a screeching halt.

Wow, I thought, what a ride, and am I glad
it was finally over. I almost expected a few
more bumps and grinds, but after a few
seconds I managed to collect my thoughts. I
couldn't see anything but blacks and grays
and tried to reach my face to focus my
glasses but they were no longer on my face.
I thought I might have lost them on the first
or second somersault I encountered, but
what did it matter if it was the first or last,
they were gone, and as I reached around to
feel for them, I noticed it was not only
Extremely cramped where I was stuffed, it
was now getting much hotter. The odors

and creaking noises caught my attention and I could feel the heat, and the smoke was starting to choke me. As would a blindman, I inched my way around in the opposite direction I felt that the heat was coming from, and after crawling over what was left of the front seat, the broken glass, the twisted metal and broken wooden parts strewn beneath my body, I felt what I thought was that cutsie little stuffed Tiger and I figured I had made it to the back window. I'm sure the flames were licking at my feet because the soles of my boots were getting pretty hot, and I knew I should get out of there as fast as Tigger [the girls named the cutsie little Tiger, Tigger] and I could before the flames came toward what was the front of my car, and reach the now cracked and spilling gas tank. I had no desire to go out in a Blaze of Glory, and I do mean Blaze. The Glory held an enchanting thought but just fleeting. I managed to crawl out of what was left of my back window and fell to the ground.

Knowing I had just filled the Stang at the base, and I only drove for about 10 miles down that Highway, it was pretty evident that I had to gather myself together and make space between the burning car and myself. I could barely see the flickering flames through the now billowing smoke, but it was too close for comfort and I could still feel the heat on my face and hands. I no sooner got to my feet when I heard an explosion and the shock blew me for what I figured was another 20-30 feet through the air. I started to get up again while wiping my face so that I could see where I was in relation to the car and the flames, but no matter how hard or how fast I wiped I just couldn`t get what I now knew was blood covering my eyes. I decided to reach around for where the blood was gushing from and found a hole in the right side of my head, above the hairline over my ear and decided to plug it up with Tigger since I felt my fingers were too small to stop the bleeding and I could kinda wiggle them in the side of my head. Thank GOD for Tigger, I thought, at least now I wouldn't bleed to death. I managed to clear most of the blood away from my eyes and tried focusing on the burning wreck to get my bearings. I had to make my way out of there, I wasn't sure where, but I figure as long as I'm walking I'm in better shape then the "Stang" was cause she wasn't going anywhere.

Just when I figure I've got things assesed pretty well: The what happened, The where was I, and conscious enough to initiated what damage control was available to me to stop most all the bleeding, I hear these Angelic Voices way off in the distance, they're calling out my name and seem to be getting louder and louder. "Lou," "Lou baby, come over here," "Come to us"...and I'm thinking...No Thank you, I've gone through enough tonight and I didn't need any more surprises. Besides, I was way too young to die and coming from a rough and tumble background I was born and raised in, I pretty well knew which direction those beautiful voices were calling me to. Hell NO, I won't go! I started thinking of the gang fights and the bar fights and all the fist fights I'd had from Brooklyn on out to Long Island and all those bars across these United States I'd been in and out of, and now I was getting ready to fight my hardest fight with the baddest dude in the Universe and I knew I wasn't ready. I needed a little more time and training for that Devil round.

I guess the funk I was in was worse than I thought because I felt these hands reaching me and pulling me in a direction I didn't think I wanted to go, but after a few of the shock waves had passed, I realized that those that were pulling me were actually holding me up, and, they were five of the girls from the party I was going to. When they noticed I hadn't shown up yet, they decided to come to the base to hurry me up so that I wouldn't miss out on that going away party, although, I almost had a more dynamic going away party just a few minutes ago, and I was sure mine was more memorable than just falling down drunk and stinking of puke. It was their Headlights I saw headed my way just prior to the crash, and they were hysterical watching this car flipping and careening down the road right before their eyes, bursting into flames. But the real Horror was when they found out it was my car. What a bummer, they went from ladies of the Night to Angels of Mercy in just a few eye opening, ear splitting, jaw dropping, breath holding minutes. All I remember them saying was "you better not die on us," and I wanted to do them that little favor so I flipped them a "thumbs up" sign. It was about all the strength I could muster by then.

They had a souped up 4dr Fairlane that they had skidded in a hasty "Huey" and had crossed the Median to reach me and the Stangs location, when they saw it finally come to a rest. Now they were trying to wisk me into the backseat of it, and rush me back to the base hospital so I could keep my promise. Three of the girls got into the back seat and the remaining two girls laid me across their laps. Then the two jumped into the frontseat and gunned that Ford toward the base as fast as they dared and believe me, they Dared. As I lay across their laps I heard one of them say through her tears, "Look, Lou saved Tigger" and when she reached for the stuffed animal she was horrified to see the blood start gushing from my head again and immediately replaced Tigger to it's lifesaving duties. Another one noticed my hand bleeding from all the glass and tore up her skirt to make a bandage. I was thinking how great these girls were for not worrying about the mess I was making on them and their car. I suddenly found myself, sort of sitting up right, looking out the back window of the speeding car, amazed at watching the burning and smoking blob that once was my "Stang" as it faded in the distance.

I felt a little cramped with my head pressed against the roof of the Fairlane and then I looked down to see the three girls crying and shouting hysterically to the driver to hurry up, when it hit me: WOW. that's me on their laps and there's nobody home! I'm looking at what was left of my poor, crumpled Mustang from out the window, and the other me is just laying there without a care. I tried to tell the girls I was alright and they could stop the crying and slow down a bit. I reached for the driver to get her attention and she turned her head slightly toward me but she seemed to be talking to the girl holding my other head and not to me because she was saying that she was going as fast as this 8 banger would go and I looked at the 110 on the speedometer and thought well hell, I could

go through another crash again, that last one
was now a piece of cake but I don't know
about that other me laying on the girls laps,
he looks in pretty bad shape even to me. I
felt no pain, no fear and I was with 5 girls
speeding down the Highway, Me and Me,
What a night so far!

It's a good thing the girls had a base sticker
on their car because the Guard at the Gate
barely had time to wave them through, they
were way ahead of him and through the
Gate in a flash, shouting to him that they
were going to the Hospital. I kinda chuckled
and waved to him out the back window as
we flew bye but he never waved back.
When we pulled up to the Hospital, both
girls in the front ran out like it was a relay
race and they hit the doors running. I started
to get out and headed for the swinging
doors when they were back already with
two corpsman and a gurney. I stepped aside
to watch them load that other me on it and
as they wisked him away, I watched the
other three girls compose themselves, and
all five headed toward the Emergency
Room. I decided to follow since no one
seemed to notice me and I wanted to see
what all the commotion was about. There
were nurses and corpsmen and a Doctor all
fussing about and a couple of the girls were
at the front desk giving information about
me to the deskclerk while the rest of them

were pressing their noses against the Operating Room windows. I walked down the corridor and looked at some of the people sitting on the benches and chairs, apparently waiting their turn to be attended to, but there was the other me at the Head of the Line, so I excused myself and headed there also.

I walked straight through the doors and walked around the doctor and nurses that were tearing off my clothes and swabbing me down. The doctor noticed the large hole in the side of my head and was cleaning it up when the corpsman that was standing toward my side asked if he could stitch up the gash on my hand. The doctor said it would be OK since He [the doctor] didn't think I would make it anyway. He said something about having to put a "Plate" in my head but that I had lost a tremendous amount of blood and didn't know if I would survive much longer. The Nurse asked if she should have the base Chaplain standby, so the Doctor lifted my dogtags. When he read "Agnostic" and Blood type "O neg." He said "I don't think this Kid would care but you can call him if you want!" I thought that was a bit insensitive, and I wasn't happy about a corpsman practicing on my hand either, and thought to myself, I should lodge a complaint, but just as those thoughts flickered past, I started to float up toward

the ceiling. It finally hit me that I could see
myself on the table being operated on
desperately and I could now see the me that
was mostly translucent floating above it all.
I looked around as I floated higher and
higher and noticed the dirt and dust on the
fluorescent lights in the OR and thought,
Some bodies gonna hear about this too,
when I heard the doc say "Tag 'N' Bag Him,
we're not going to need that plate nurse.
Corpman, are you done on that hand?" "Yes
Sir, he replied and the Doctor said: "Fine,
sheet him for now son." I knew what was
going on just then to the me I knew, but I
wasn't ready for what was about to happen
to the Me I now was.

I was about to attempt to reach the girls that
were now crying and hugging each other
but instead of going forward, I was being
pulled backward and upward. I had no sense
of fear, none of loss, actually all I felt was
wonderment and curiosity and anticipation
of what was to come.

I entered what I thought looked like the
Holland tunnel, without the cars and traffic,
and the ability to see what looked like light
at it's end. It was dark but not black, the
path was slightly illuminated from what I
thought to be the Sunlight shining from the
other end. As I was being drawn toward the
lighted end of the Tunnel, I carefully looked

around, even squinting to see into the darker recesses. I passed what I thought to be very religious men doing what they would do when praying to their GODS. They were all dressed in their finest garbs, robes, togas, head dresses, loin cloths and the like. Most of them were off to the sides of the tunnel, but one of them, that I seemed to float right over, looked oriental with a long grayish Fu Man Chu, sitting there in the middle of the tunnel, with his hands clasped and his feet crossed. Since I had just completed two tours "In Country" I figured he must represent the last of the religions I sought to make my own. I was raised Catholic but withdrew from that faith at an early age and delved into many others from the Mayan to Koran to Hopi as well as all North and South American Native beliefs. It looked like they were all represented here. When I floated past the monk just below me, I thought he could actually see me because it appeared like he began to smile a smile of passage. All the other Religious men were mumbling sounds of prayer and were moving their arms about as if making gestures of a Blessing. I wasn't sure if they were Blessing me or the Tunnel. I noticed none of them were actually standing or sitting in the Tunnel but appeared to be levitated. I wanted to stop and speak with some of them, maybe ask a few questions like who they were and how long have they

been here, but I was being wisked away
toward the Light. I saw wisps of smoke I
believed to be incense, it came from all
portions of the Great Tunnel from one end
to the other. I could see and smell but I had
not yet had the sensation of touch since my
feet were never touching the tunnels floor
and I seemed to be traveling squarely in the
center as I drifted toward the end. The
closer I got to the end of the Tunnel, the
brighter things got, and as I neared the end,
it was like coming face to face with a huge
canvas that was just recently blazed in the
brightest white of whites. An empty canvas,
ready to be painted upon and I awaited that
painting. Then in an instant, my entire life,
starting from birth through the present was
flashing before my eyes like a strobe light at
half speed. Frame after frame, some parts in
freeze frame, if only for a second, then on
to the next. I felt as if I was being subjected
to a test to see if this was in fact the me that
was supposed to be here and then it ended
as fast as it had begun. The last scene was
that of a rolling mass of metal finally
bursting into flames, and I was looking at
the canvas again.

While staring into the vast whiteness I
glanced down to look at my body and use it
for a reference, only to find the translucent
outline I once had was no longer there. I
thought, How could this be? Am I now part

of this empty white canvas, but if I were,
then where are my thoughts coming from to
be asking these questions. Instantly I
recognized a brilliant glowing ball of gold
headed my way. It grew larger as it grew
nearer and when it reached about the size of
a beachball, just above and in front of me it
radiated brilliantly and transformed into an
indescribable Being of pure LIGHT, now
levitated right in front of me. It was larger
than the tallest person I had ever seen,
wider than two of me, but so evenly
proportioned as to be of Magnificent
Stature. It's features were outlined as if
made with a fine ink quill. Hair, face, robe
all Golden and flowing as would an electric
charge perhaps even a nuclear charge. This
was energy personifide and as it's form took
on a more solid shape, all that was behind It
did as well. It was as if the Entire canvas of
white I had come to at the end of the Tunnel
was now alive and I was part of it. Other
figures appeared in front and behind the
Being and myself. Soon there was activity
all about, above and below, on every side,
more beings, each of different brightness,
sizes, and hues. Structures and landscapes
sprung from everywhere all in a crystalline
state, all inhabited by these lesser light
beings, some winged, most not, Some fully
formed, others not, yet even others that
appeared only as glowing Orbs of light and

color, bouncing as would bubbles in a glass
of carbonated water.

I could stand it no longer, every emotion I
had ever known was welling up in me ten-
fold. Just when I thought to speak, to
question, the Being spoke to me. It's voice
was as a chorus of voices, not male nor
female, not loud nor soft, not deep but
perfect and all encomposing. As I looked at
the two gigantic, magnificent beings
dressed in Brilliant capes just off to IT's
side, IT said, "that is Michael and Gabrial.
Michael has chosen you as his and Gabrial
shall teach you the ways." I looked past
them to another Large Being, so beautiful
but darker in contrast, as was the sprawling
robe it wore. This being had eyes that
pleased but pierced with it's gaze, and the
Light Being said "that is He who has been
cast out. You who I have given choice may
go with any of these of your choosing." I
thought as I had a choice, and Michael had
already chosen me then I would chose Him.
He appeared so strong and mighty, as did
the others, but in his eyes seemed a fire that
was drawing and captivating to me.
Gabrials eyes were softer and gave more in
an understanding manner and I thought "Oh
how absolutely Beautiful are these Beings."
I then looked to The Being before me and
It's eyes were full of Love and warmth,
authoritative and compelling. He seemed to

have approved of my choice, Then said to me "You will be my soldier and you will go with Michael for a while. Gabrial will come to you at times. I will send others to you and your fruit shall not fall far from from the tree in the time of the Gathering."

Just then I saw five Orbs of Light. They seemed to be playing, swirling round and about the Being and myself. They had appeared from the outlying landscape and I noticed they were all the same size and shape but of different hues as subtle as shades of rose petals, save one which had a bluish hue. Two of the pinkish ones seemed exactly alike, the other two were yet deeper in shades of red and orange, and before I could ask, IT spoke and said "They, like all here are of you, who are of me, but these will come to you and you will care for them more. They will fly apart but come together at the time of the Gathering." I thought The Being might be telling me these were my children but I was only 21 and not only had never been married but had no plans to. I didn't understand how all this was of me and me of HE when a magnificent crystal serving platter appeared and it shimmered the colors of many rainbows. In an instant it shattered into thousands of pieces, each piece brilliant in its own right. Ever so slowly now all the pieces began to rejoin themselves to once again form the original

serving platter once again and I now knew
what this Being of Light was showing me,
we pieces are the platter. I was just one of
those thousands of pieces, as were all those
I was seeing here and those back in the
"World." Now my mind was still trying to
ponder The Gathering. As I thought what
could this mean, The Being answered,
"Here you will see the signs that bring forth
the Gathering," and with that I saw frames
appear like screens on a TV set. When I
looked into the screens, the visions would
gather up, pop off in an image, and enter
my mind. I felt as if I was being pushed
back with it's impact. They were only
glimpses but they were so realistic, as if
happening right there in front of me in the
now. I could not turn away and then it
seemed that I had become a part of each of
these visions. There were scenes of men in
uniform killing other men in uniforms, I
recognized some of the insignias and some
were from the USA. There were also
thousands of them not in uniforms killing
even more thousands not in uniform. It was
like looking at toy figures moving on their
own, mowing down other figures, different
countries, different Nations, different
Religions, different weapons, different
Decades, but always resulting in hundreds
of thousands dead and dying. I wanted out
of there, I could feel the pain these people
were suffering. I asked the Being why was

this, and how long was this to go on, and
The Being said "Man will prey on man,
Until Man will pray for man".

The next vision was of floods, many of
them spilling across the Earth on different
continents in different seasons and I am
again walking among it, feeling the force
and taking in the smell of Death. Hundreds
of Lives and acres upon acres of crops were
lost as well as hundreds of stock and wild
animals floating away into the abiss. Then I
was watching Volcanoes from around the
world erupting, first one then another. The
molten Lava burying whole towns and
villages and the people and animals within
them. I gazed among the ruins and saw little
left of what once stood there. The last
vision I saw in the screen were of
Earthquakes destroying sections of almost
every continent. One was a masssive one in
America, most others were in Europe and
the Orient. Again thousands are killed,
structures are crumpled, the landscape
leveled and I turned again to the Being and
He said "There will not only be more of
what you have seen but there will come a
time when it will all happen at the same
time and it will come at the same time of
mans greatest sins." I didn't have time to
ask, when HE said "They will turn from ME
and claim themselves like Gods." With that
Michael beckons me to go with him and I

am now part of the Universe. Novas, Suns, Planets, all that I looked at from the Earth, not so long ago, or was it?

We traveled toward the beginning of it all, the inner portions of the Universe. Kazillions of planets around Kazillions of Suns and the closer to the center we approached the more concentrated the number of Galaxies. It is like the Plate you saw, the largest part, after it shattered was at the center and those parts that shattered first were sent the farthest from the center, So is everything in the Universe. All is but a circle within a circle wrapped in a circle. Each level, each dimension is but a layer of the original which is without end. I watched as millions of Orbs systematically entered the many Planets before me. They appeared as Bees flitting from flower to flower, pollinating each, one after another. Michael took me closer and I could now see that so many of these Planets had life on them and the Orbs were joining with the creatures of these Planets. Not every Creature was the same on every Planet but they all had some commonalities, a head, a body, extremities and the Light Beings would animate them for a time. We headed away from the center now and Michael said that Gabrial would have more to explain to me and that He, Michael, wanted me to know that He was pleased with the many times He had called

on me to do His bidding and that I
performed my duties well. His parting
words were "You will never again be made
to forget!"

I was journeying back to where I knew
Earth would be and watched as Comets and
Asteriods casually passed by me or I passed
them. The colors of the gasious cloud
formations were striking. I started looking
at these infant galaxies as one would cloud
formations back on Earth, imagining what
shape they were taking on, This one a boat,
this a bird with wings, this a scarf floating
in the breeze, till I recogonized what was
the Constellation ORION and I knew I was
getting close to my destination. While
drifting through ORION, I noticed two
Blazing Celestial Bodies racing parallel to
it's center, looking as Twin Arrows exiting
from an Archers Bow and headed straight
for the "Blue Marble" of home.
Immediately a vision of Millions of people
crying because of the devastation of
portions of New York City came to me. I
became aware of a strange feeling I had not
known previously, and I thought that might
be because this was the city I had grown up
in. I saw a huge Earthquake, a magnitude of
8.6 in someplace named EUREKA. A ham
operator or radio announcer was directing
thousands of people migrating from areas of
frequent disasters to places of safety. A

space station appeared to be falling from the heavens because of an internal explosion. Missles were being simutaniously fired into space from several Nations. I thought the Light Being had shown me all there was to see but these were different, stronger and there was no pre-screening as before. Gabrial appeared beside me, I thought because I had felt shaky, but it was to explain the now sprawling Galatic View of my Galaxy.

The Sun was expanding and spewing off Huge ecto-plasma balls, more then it has ever done in it's past, and in the very direction the Planets would orbit through. I could not take my eyes from the Earth and as I watched what effect these eruptions would have on the Earth, A large Mass passed me, larger than any of the Planets known to me, and as it passes, I see the Earth wobble wildly as would a top toward the end of its spin. The rotation stopped and slowly started again but it was tilted now and I was drawn in closer like the zoom of a lens. The ash clouds that had engulfed the Earth thinned, and like a tack welded piece of metal being dismantled, I could see the Ocean bodies starting to rise, first the Pacific, along the "Ring of Fire", then the others, syncretisticly. As the waters shifted upon the landmasses, the landmasses started to sink under the waters added pressure upon it. When the pressures equaled out to the spin of the changing axis, the Earth no longer looked as it did moments before. It was newer, cleaner, more beautiful with darker Greens and lighter Blues. Some of the new landmasses looked similar to a few of the other Planets I had recently visited with Michael. People were upon this Earth and appeared happier and more content although seemingly living like the Native populations of old. Cities, built by the Ancient Ones, that were buried beneath the Oceans were now being populated by the surviving people in this new world. I saw Tribes joining tribes and small Nations forming, but it was what I didn't see that made my heart glow, there were no more wars, true peace and happiness had finally befallen on mankind. Gabrial now tells me that this is His message that I must take back, to let others know that there is little to fear, for the Earth will go on forever, as did all the Planets I had visited. I am to tell the world to look to ORION, and they will know when the new world will come upon them. I ask Him "What of the others there on Earth, during the change?" Gabrial tells me that all will be lifted, some will be lifted higher than others and no longer enjoy the physical plane, while some will be left on the Earth to replenish and rebuild the physical, they too will be of a higher elevation then any that are living there now!

I was now before the Light Being of Gold
again, those five orbs were still darting
about. I wanted to stay and explore this
realm with all the other light beings but I
was told I could not. I was brought here to
go back to tell the others who would be
coming after me, that if they would spread
the Love they brought with them to the
physical world they would know their
Creator eagerly awaits them. The Being told
me that should I ever have questions of the
heart or mind, that He will answer them, if I
only look within myself, for that is where
He will dwell. From this time forward I
need only think it to be so and it will be so
for I would forever know the truth. I was
told there was much work left undone and
that He had set a road of rocks before me
that I must sweep away for passage. Many
will be set before me that I may help in my
presence, and more I will not, but that I
must not set aside wrongly, for a soul
should not be lost within my heart. I asked
how I would know and before I received an
answer I was being wisked away through
that darkened tunnel like a dust bunny in a
vacuum, with about as much control as a
runaway freight train.

I awoke to a nurse scrubbing the encrusted
blood off of the right side of my head. My
body was racked with pain. I screamed at
the nurse for what I felt was her lack of

compassion and she had a shocked look on her face. "Oh my God, Welcome back sailor. We thought you were a goner for sure." I asked her where was I and how long had I been here and she answered: "You've been in a coma for seven days now. They thought you died on the operating table and was going to ship you to the Morgue when the assisting corpsman noticed some movement under your sheet and rushed you back to the OR. The doctor checked you out and he was amazed to find your vitals were returning to normal but what really floored him was the hardened crust that had formed over the hole in your head seemed to have sealed most of the damage. He decided he didn`t even have to put a steel plate in your head any more as it had healed sufficently on it's own in the time you were gone." I said "you mean that practicing corpman that was sewing my hand in the operating room saved my life?" She said "Yes, but how did you know he was sewing your hand? You were unconscious the entire time you were in OR and never came to until just now." If she had only known all the things I knew from that time she would have surely gone in to shock. I took the brush and towel from her hands and said I would finish the job for her and she thanked me and said she was going to notify the doctors that I was alive and conscious!

I looked across the dorm and saw several sailors and a Marine lying in their perspective beds. The Marine looked familiar and was situated closest to me. He smiled and said "Hey, Mr. Chuck [a handle I picked up overseas] You missed a hellava party last week." I replied "So I am told," but you should have seen the one I went to, it was a real mind blower." He told me I made the local papers and a picture of what was left of my car was photographed and on the 2nd page of the news. Then he said "I bet you're glad they are going to sign your discharge papers and not your Death Certificate like they almost did." I joked and said "yeah, you know those Navy doctors, in and out, they'd sign anything to get their Liberty passes." The doctor finally arrived and started to check me out. He seemed genuinely interested yet amazed at my seemingly miraculous recovery. He checked the side of my head first, then ran his hands over my arms and legs. He asked if I could stand after giving me the "follow my fingers and how many are there" doctor thing. I jumped out of bed and he stood agast. He asked if I could raise my arms over my head[thinking I could not] and when I did he asked if I could slowly reach my toes [which I did] and then he sat me on the bed and started to talk to me. He told me I was a medical miracle. Not only was I not supposed to still be alive after the massive

blood loss, but the mental trauma of my
head injury would at the least make me a
vegetable. He also said that the injuries to
my legs and arms alone should have kept
me in the infirmary for another two to three
weeks. Yet there I was, everything working
fine, actually as good as new, not even any
black and blue marks to show what my
body had been through. He said he had to
admit it was truly a marvel and when I
askcd if I could bc rcturned to Active Duty,
he said he really couldn't see why not. He
signed my hospital discharge papers and I
was returned to my Squad the next day.

It was good to be among the living but I
knew it was a far, far, better place I had
been, than any place here on Earth will ever
be again. I remembered everything that
happened to me in that other place but
spoke none of it to anyone because just the
mention of having been dead was enough to
make people twirl their fingers near their
brain when they thought I wasn't looking,
and some times I wasn't looking, but I
knew!

L. F.

A Suicide Story

Just wanted to relate a suicide story.

I know that this world is especially tough on our young people right now, and that there are those young people who consider suicide as a way out, I know, I was one. After you read this story I hope you will realize how foolish and self centered it is.

This story is about a 17-year-old high school youth named Tom. He lived across the street with his family from my best friend in the mid-1980's. He had been doing some PCP (a popular, and very dangerous drug) and it really messed him up psychologically. He was being treated for some months with anti-depressants.

On the first day that he stopped taking them he went into his parent's bedroom (where there was a cabinet of his step-father's guns, him being a cop) and shot himself. Apparently he was very resentful of his mother re-marrying and was always acting out, not able to just accept it. His mother had already gone to work for the day so he thought that he was alone at the time. His 8-year-old sister was late going to school and heard the shot and discovered him.

She called her mother at work and the
mother came home to find him, dying. Two
days later I went over with my friend with
some food to visit with her. I notice while
we were sitting with her (I was sitting
across from her) that there was this flash
that streaked toward her on her right side. I
thought that this was odd and began
thinking about what this could mean later
after we had left.

When I really looked at that light what I
saw was her son, Tom, racing toward her
repeatedly, desperate to get her attention.
He was in such agony, because he needed to
tell his mother how sorry he was. He
thought that by killing himself that he could
just be out of pain and that all his problems
would be solved. Now he was in his own
private hell of his own making and there
was no way to stop it.

I can still to this day feel his agony and
shock that he was not able to communicate
with his mother when he was right there,
she couldn't notice him. He was so very
terrified, he didn't know what else to do.
When you die, even by your own hand, you
are still conscious, you still know what is
going on but are helpless to do anything
about it so it makes your problems even
worse.

Just do what you have to do to get help.
When you are young, you feel like your
problems are so permanent that there is
nothing that you can do. Don't believe it,
there is always something that you can do.
There is always a way out, don't give up,
your life is worth everything. May God
Bless the young people of this world, you
have value or you wouldn't be in this world!

J.W.

About the Author

The author didn't write anything until after fifty. For over 40 years he worked in the "words-on-paper" business. Printing and typesetting his way through life. He owned a small typesetting business until computers took over. What prompted him to write web pages, blogs and books was a heart attack. At the age of 49 he suffered a strong heart attack which lead to a Near Death Experience. This event changed his perspective of life and opened a whole new world to investigate. After considerable research he began to write about spiritual subjects. Discovering the vast difference between religion and spirituality was like finding a peace and calm never before known to him.

Then his writing turned to poetry which seemed a natural progression for him. Some poems were a struggle and others rolled off his pen as fast as he could write like they were dictated by someone unseen. The poetry is widely varied. Some spiritual, some humorous, and some will touch your heart. A few poems came from the personal experiences of the author, others just good thoughts for living a better life.

...and Finally

God loves you more than you realize, more than you
can imagine while in physical form. He sets no limits or
conditions. His Love is unconditional. You don't have
to do anything, believe anything, or be anyone special
to deserve it. You are His perfect child.

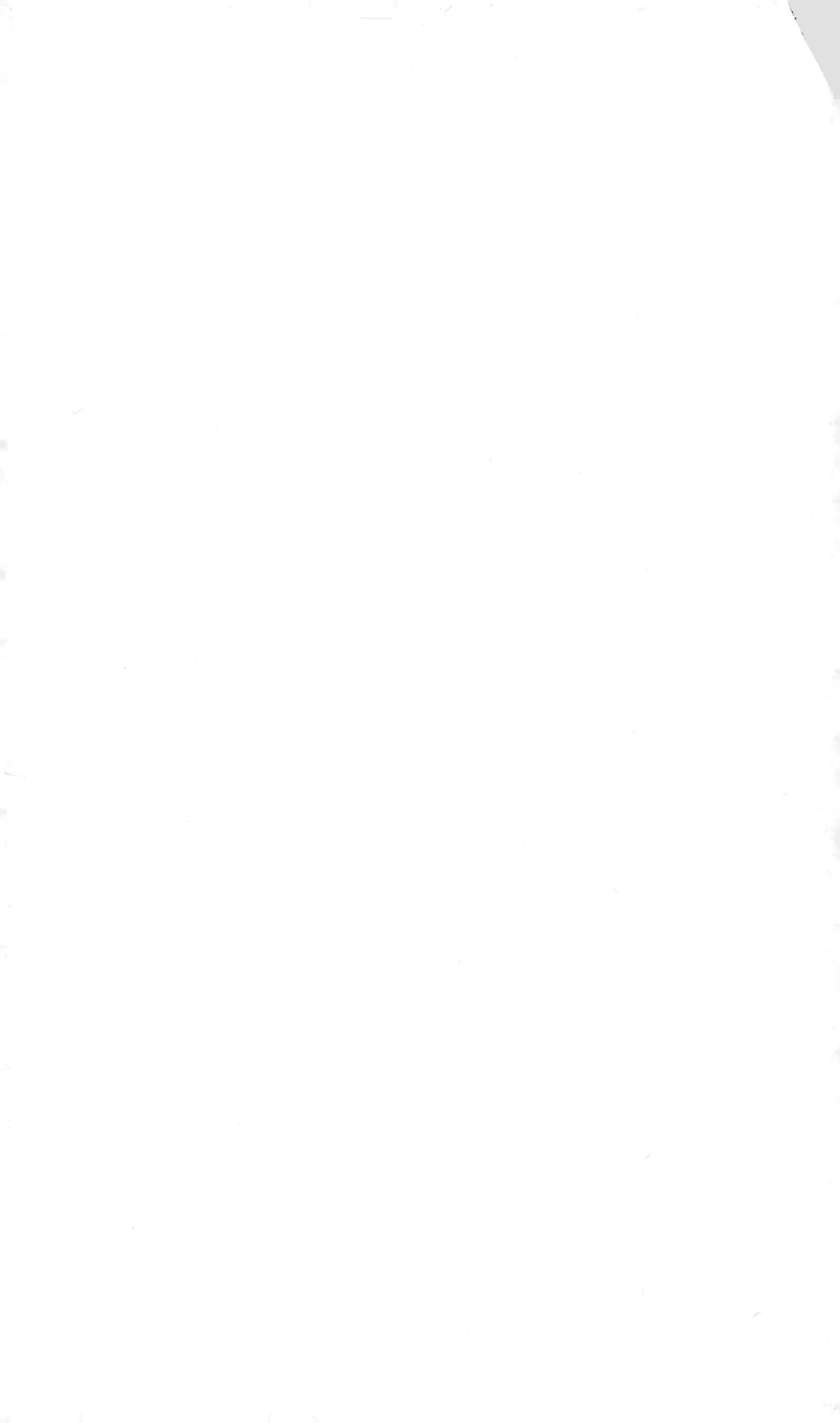

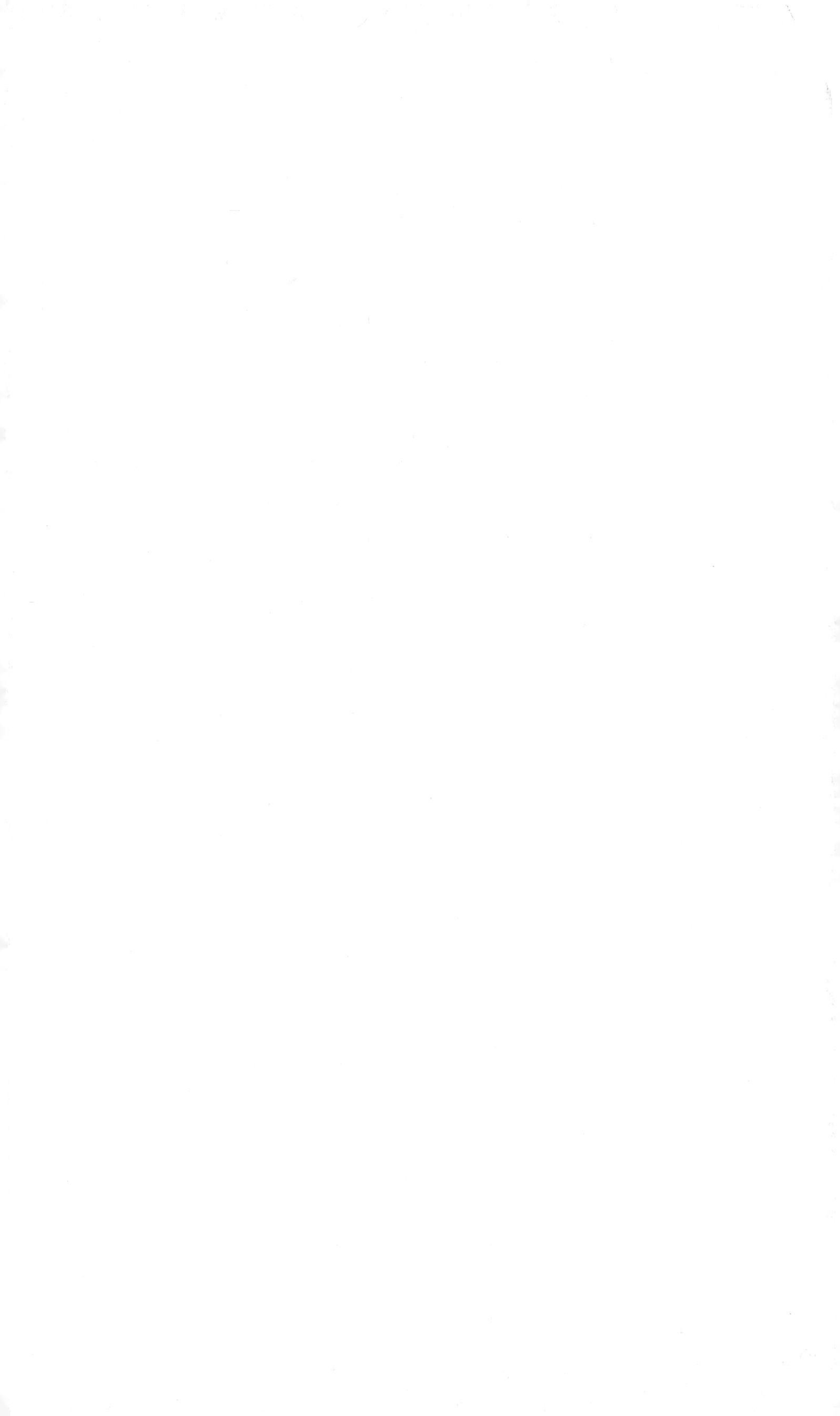

www.ingramcontent.com/pod-product-compliance
Lightning Source LLC
Chambersburg PA
CBHW061621250726
48659CB00004B/1037